INVASOMES AS DRUG NANOCARRIERS FOR INNOVATIVE PHARMACEUTICAL DOSAGE FORMS

INVASOMES AS DRUG NANOCARRIERS FOR INNOVATIVE PHARMACEUTICAL DOSAGE FORMS

Nina Dragićević
Associate Professor
Department of Pharmacy
Singidunum University
Belgrade, Serbia

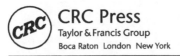
CRC Press
Taylor & Francis Group
Boca Raton London New York

CRC Press is an imprint of the
Taylor & Francis Group, an **informa** business

First edition published 2021
by CRC Press
6000 Broken Sound Parkway NW, Suite 300, Boca Raton, FL 33487-2742

and by CRC Press
2 Park Square, Milton Park, Abingdon, Oxon, OX14 4RN

© 2021 Taylor & Francis Group, LLC

CRC Press is an imprint of Taylor & Francis Group, LLC

Library of Congress Cataloging-in-Publication Data
Names: Dragicevic, Nina, author.
Title: Invasomes as drug nanocarriers for innovative pharmaceutical dosage forms / Nina Dragićević.
Description: First edition. | Boca Raton : CRC Press, 2021. | Includes bibliographical references and index. | Summary: "This book details the novel nanocarriers named 'invasomes' and how they are used for dermal and transdermal drug delivery. The text describes their composition, usage of skin as a drug delivery route and liposomes as skin delivery systems. Included are reviewed studies revealing the importance of invasomes in this field"-- Provided by publisher.
Identifiers: LCCN 2021031149 (print) | LCCN 2021031150 (ebook) | ISBN 9781032028651 (hardback) | ISBN 9781032034515 (paperback) | ISBN 9781003187332 (ebook)
Subjects: LCSH: Drug delivery systems. | Nanomedicine. | Skin absorption. | Transdermal medication. | Liposomes.
Classification: LCC RS199.5 .D693 2021 (print) | LCC RS199.5 (ebook) | DDC 615.1/9--dc23
LC record available at https://lccn.loc.gov/2021031149
LC ebook record available at https://lccn.loc.gov/2021031150

ISBN: 978-1-032-02865-1 (hbk)
ISBN: 978-1-032-03451-5 (pbk)
ISBN: 978-1-003-18733-2 (ebk)

DOI: 10.1201/9781003187332

Typeset in Times
by MPS Limited, Dehradun

Contents

Preface   ix
About the Author   xi

1 The Skin as a Drug Delivery Route   **1**
1.1   Introduction   1
1.2   The Skin   2
       1.2.1   Epidermis   2
               1.2.1.1   The stratum corneum – primary
                         permeability barrier   3
1.3   Dermal and Transdermal Drug Delivery   8
       1.3.1   Therapeutic Target Sites in Dermal and
               Transdermal Delivery   8
       1.3.2   Advantages of Dermal and Transdermal Drug
               Delivery   10
1.4   Drug Transport Routes Through the Skin   14
1.5   Factors Affecting Drug Permeation Rate Through
       the Skin   18
1.6   Penetration Enhancement Techniques-classification   19
       1.6.1   Chemical Penetration Enhancers   19
1.7   Conclusion   22

**2 Lipid-Based Vesicles (Liposomes) as Skin Delivery
Systems**   **31**
2.1   Composition and Classification of Liposomes   31
       2.1.1   Physicochemical Properties of Liposomes
               Influencing their Penetration-Enhancing
               Ability   35
2.2   Liposomes as Skin Drug Delivery Systems   43
       2.2.1   Liposomes as Topical Drug Delivery Systems
               (Localizing Effects)   43
       2.2.2   Liposomes as Drug Delivery Systems
               Targeting the Skin Appendages   44

                                                                               v

2.3   Novel Vesicles as Transdermal Drug Delivery Systems   57
      2.3.1   Transfersomes   58
2.4   Mechanisms of Action of Liposomes/vesicles   72
      2.4.1   Penetration of Intact Liposomes/Vesicles   72
      2.4.2   Penetration-Enhancing Mechanism of
              Vesicles' Components and Vesicle
              Adsorption to and/or Fusion With SC Lipids   90
      2.4.3   Free Drug Process – Penetration of the Drug
              Released From Vesicles   93
2.5   Conclusion   94

3 **Invasomes for Dermal and Transdermal Drug Delivery**   **109**
3.1   Development of Invasomes   109
3.2   Terpenes as Penetration Enhancers Enclosed in
      Invasomes   111
      3.2.1   Structure-Activity Relationship of Terpenes   113
      3.2.2   Lipophilicity of the Drug   114
      3.2.3   Mechanism of Skin Penetration
              Enhancement by Terpenes   115
      3.2.4   Synergistic Action of Terpenes with Co-Solvents   118
3.3   Ethanol   119
3.4   Preparation, Physico-chemical Properties and Stability
      of Invasomes   122
      3.4.1   Preparation of Invasomes   122
      3.4.2   Characterization of Invasomes   123
3.5   Invasomes as Penetration Enhancers   129
      3.5.1   Enhanced Percutaneous Penetration of
              Immunosuppresive Drugs   131
      3.5.2   Enhanced Percutaneous Penetration of
              Photosensitizers   141
      3.5.3   Enhanced Percutaneous Penetration of
              Hydrophilic Model Drugs   145
      3.5.4   Enhanced Percutaneous Penetration of Skin
              Lighteners   147
      3.5.5   Enhanced Percutaneous Penetration of
              Antioxidants   148
      3.5.6   Enhanced Percutaneous Penetration of Drugs
              for the Management of Prostatic Hyperplasia   149
      3.5.7   Enhanced Percutaneous Penetration of
              Curcumin   151

	3.5.8	Enhanced Percutaneous Penetration of Antihypertensive Drugs	152
	3.5.9	Enhanced Percutaneous Penetration of Isotretinoin for the Treatment of Eosinophilic Pustular Folliculitis	156
	3.5.10	Enhanced Percutaneous Penetration of Nonsteroidal Anti-Inflammatory Drugs	156
	3.5.11	Enhanced Percutaneous Penetration of Drugs for the Treatment of Acne Vulgaris	158
	3.5.12	Enhanced Percutaneous Penetration of Drugs for the Treatment of *Alopecia*	159
	3.5.13	Enhanced Percutaneous Penetration of Drugs for the Treatment of Erectile Dysfunction	160
3.6	Invasomes as Penetration Enhancers Combined With Physical Penetration Enhancing Methods		162
	3.6.1	Invasomes Combined with Microneedles	162
	3.6.2	Invasomes Combined with Ultrasound	167
	3.6.3	Invasomes Combined with Massage	170
3.7	*In vivo* and *In Vitro* Therapeutic Effectiveness of Invasomes		171
	3.7.1	Invasomes in the Treatment of Alopecia Areata	171
	3.7.2	Invasomes in Photodynamic Therapy and Anti-Cancer Therapy	174
	3.7.3	Invasomes in Treatment of *Acne Vulgaris*	176
	3.7.4	Invasomes in the Treatment of Hypertension	179
	3.7.5	Invasomes for Skin Lightening	180
	3.7.6	Invasomes in Treatment of Bacterial Infections	180
3.8	Fluidity of Invasomes		181
3.9	Mode of Action of Invasomes		184
3.10	The Safety Profile of Invasomes		186
3.11	Conclusion		188
Index			207

Preface

The aim of this unique, peer-reviewed volume is to provide to readers in academia and industry, including young researchers, an up-to-date comprehensive work describing all topics required to understand the principles of enhancing transdermal and dermal drug delivery by the novel phospholipid-based vesicles named *invasomes*. The book is divided into three chapters.

The first chapter begins with a description of the skin with emphasis on the stratum corneum, representing its uppermost layer which is responsible for barrier function. Understanding the structure, function and especially penetration pathways is fundamental to learning how topical and transdermal drug delivery systems work and how different methods may be employed to enhance percutaneous drug penetration. The advantages of dermal and transdermal drug delivery systems are described, as well as properties of drugs required for their efficient penetration into/through the skin, and a list of possible penetration enhancement methods used to overcome the impermeability of the skin barrier. Nanocarriers are presented and these are a means for the percutaneous penetration enhancement of drugs.

The second chapter is devoted to the development of phospholipid-based vesicles, i.e. liposomes, their role as nanocarriers, being mostly used as topical drug delivery systems (for localized effects in the skin) and drug delivery systems targeting the skin appendages, as well as their mechanism of penetration enhancement. Nowadays it is generally believed that conventional liposomes are of little or no value as carriers for transdermal drug delivery, as they do not penetrate deeply into the skin but rather remain at the upper layers of the stratum corneum. There was a need to develop a new generation of lipid-based vesicles, the so-called elastic/deformable vesicles, such as the invasomes and other vesicles.

After providing information on liposomes in the second chapter as being fundamental to understanding how lipid vesicles, generally, are formed and act as nanocarriers, the third chapter introduces the potent new elastic vesicles termed invasomes which contain small amounts of terpenes and ethanol, besides phospholipids and aqueous phase. The chapter gives a detailed description of invasomes development, physico-chemical characterization, stability, possible mechanism of action, their role as nanocarriers for dermal and transdermal delivery of a variety of drugs and their *in vitro* and *in vivo* therapeutic effectiveness. The numerous studies described in the chapter confirmed their promising role as nanocarriers for both dermal and transdermal drug delivery. The chapter ends with the current status and future perspectives of invasomes as potent dermal and transdermal drug delivery systems.

We are very thankful to our collaborators from Taylor & Francis, Hilary Lafoe, Danielle Zarfati and the team for their dedicated work, which was necessary to achieve a high standard of publication.

Nina Dragićević

About the Author

Dr. Nina Dragićević is Associate Professor at the Department of Pharmacy, Singidunum University in Belgrade, Serbia. She graduated from the University of Belgrade, Faculty of Pharmacy, in 1999. Subsequently she earned a Magister Degree and a PhD (*summa cum laude*, Dr. rer. nat.) in pharmaceutical technology from the University of Belgrade, Serbia and the Friedrich-Schiller University Jena, Germany, respectively. Earlier, Dr. Dragićević worked as an accredited specialist in pharmaceutical technology in the state pharmaceutical chain Apoteka "Beograd" in Belgrade. From 2007 to 2013, she was responsible for the preparation of compounded drugs for different routes of administration in pharmacies of Apoteka "Beograd", while from 2013 to 2017 she was appointed Director of the Production Department in the same company. She has published in a variety of international journals and she was the editor of six books.

The Skin as a Drug Delivery Route

1

1.1 INTRODUCTION

The skin is the largest organ in humans which covers the whole body. The total area of the skin is about 1.8 m^2 in the average-sized adult man and 1.6 m^2 in the average-sized woman. The primary function of the skin is to provide a barrier between the body and the external environment, protecting the body against chemicals, microorganisms, loss of moisture and body nutrients, and permeation of ultraviolet radiation. The skin has a role in homeostasis, i.e. in the regulation of body temperature and blood pressure, etc. Besides having these roles, the skin has also become recognized in the past three to four decades as an important drug delivery route. The skin is the most accessible organ in the body, thus, can be reached directly. Therefore, there is considerable interest in the skin as a site of drug application for achieving both *local (topical)* and *systemic (transdermal) effects*, the first used in the treatment of different skin diseases and the latter as an alternative route for systemic drug administration. However, despite being an ideal site for the application of different *dermal* and *transdermal drug formulations*, the skin represents a formidable barrier to the penetration/permeation of compounds into/through the skin. In order to develop efficient methods able to circumvent this permeation barrier, it is of crucial importance to understand the structure and function of the skin, its penetration pathways, as well as drug properties important for its percutaneous penetration.

DOI: 10.1201/9781003187332-1

1.2 THE SKIN

The skin acts as a barrier for the diffusion of substances into the underlying tissue (Schaefer and Redelmeier, 1996; Bouwstra et al., 2003). Thus, the main problem in dermal and transdermal administration of drugs is overcoming this natural barrier (Barry, 2001; Bouwstra et al., 2003). The skin is composed of anatomically distinct layers: *epidermis, dermis and subcutaneous layer – hipodermis*. In addition, there are appendageal features including hair follicles and eccrine and apocrine sweat ducts that traverse various skin layers (Figure 1.1).

1.2.1 Epidermis

The *epidermis* is composed of the *stratum corneum* (10–20 μm thick) and the underlying *viable epidermis* (50–100 μm), which consists of *stratum granulosum, stratum spinosum* and *stratum basale*. There is also an additional layer, the *stratum lucidum* (clear layer), which can be observed on parts of the body with thickened skin, such as the palm and sole of the foot. The *stratum lucidum* is often considered as the lower part of the *stratum corneum*. The viable epidermis is responsible for the generation of the *stratum corneum* through

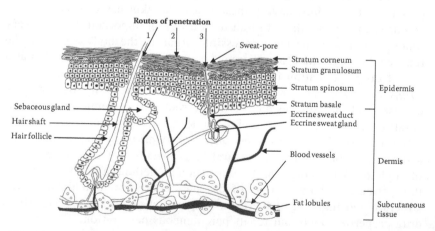

FIGURE 1.1 Simplified diagram of the skin structure and macroroutes of drug penetration: (1) through the hair follicles with their associated sebaceous glands, (2) across the continuous stratum corneum or (3) through sweat ducts. Modified from Williams (2003).

keratinocyte differentiation. Except *stratum corneum*, the rest of the epidermis is composed of nucleated cells, and is therefore termed as *viable epidermis* (Schaefer and Redelmeier, 1996). Since the *stratum corneum* provides the primary barrier of the skin, it will be discussed here in detail, while for other epidermis layers, dermis and hypodermis, the reader should refer to Schaefer and Redelmeier (1996).

1.2.1.1 The Stratum Corneum – Primary Permeability Barrier

The *stratum corneum* (horny layer, SC) is the outermost layer of the skin. It is the final product of keratinocyte differentiation (cornification). It is made of about 20 layers of metabolically inactive cells, embedded in an extracellular matrix of lamellar lipid bilayers. Corneocytes provide the physical and chemical stability of the SC, while the extracellular matrix gives it the rigid structure, impermeable barrier for water and water-soluble compounds. The SC can be considered as a wall consisting of polyhedric squeeze-protein "bricks" and water-depleted stiff lipid sheets as "mortar" (Elias, 1983). The protection of the skin is provided primarily by the SC, which due to its specific structure provides the primary barrier to percutaneous absorption of compounds as well as to water loss (Lindberg and Forslind, 2000; Bouwstra et al., 2003). In addition to the *stratum corneum*, recent findings showed that the viable epidermis is also a rate-limiting barrier to drug penetration (Andrews et al., 2012).

Corneocytes arise in the cornification process and represent cell remnants of terminally differentiated keratinocytes of the viable epidermis. The cornification process is accompanied by: the gradual loss of subcellular organelles (nucleus and cytoplasmic membrane structures) in the outermost cells of the granular layer, fusion of keratohyalin granules with keratin filament bundles and the discharge of lamellar granule contents into the intercellular space. Following this, the cells become transformed into dead, flattened, anucleate, keratinized cells of the SC. Within the corneocytes remains only the tightly packed raft of keratin fibrils (80% of total dry mass of corneocytes) oriented parallel to the long dimension of the cell with some associated filaggrin. Between the keratin fibers is a matrix consisting of the remains of keratohyalin. The protein composition of corneocytes is highly structured, insoluble and exhibits considerable resistance to chemical and physical denaturation, which contributes to its role in skin protection (Schaefer and Redelmeier, 1996; Downing and Stewart, 2000; Williams, 2003). In addition, during the cornification process, the corneocyte protein envelope is added between the internal surface of the cell membrane and the stacks of keratin fibers (Downing and Stewart, 2000). The cornified envelope is insoluble and more resistant to attempts at solubilization than the core proteins. This can be attributed to the fact that the cornified envelope is stabilized through the high degree of cross-linking of core proteins (90% of its dry mass) to the envelope and through covalently bound lipid (10% of its dry mass) (Schaefer and Redelmeier, 1996). Hence, it consists of two layers. The layer adjacent to the cytoplasm is thick and composed of structural proteins, i.e. involucrin, elafin, small proline-rich proteins, loricrin, filaggrin and keratin intermediate filaments. The layer on the exterior of the protein layer is composed of lipids. It is proposed that hydroxyceramide molecules from the lipid layer attach to the glutamate-rich protein involucrin in the cornified envelope. Thus, the lipid layer provides an anchor to the keratinocyte and links the proteinaceous domains to the intercellular lipid domains. In addition, corneocytes are joined by protein "rivets", corneodesmosomes, which contribute to the mechanical strength of the viable epidermis by effectively crosslinking the corneocytes (Schaefer and Redelmeier, 1996; Downing and Lazo, 2000; Williams, 2003).

Intercellular lipids account for approximately only 15% of the dry weight of the SC, but play an important role in the cohesion of the SC. They are derived from the terminally differentiated keratinocytes, i.e. from the lamellar bodies which are discharged during the differentiation. The differentiation process of keratinocytes is accompanied by dramatic changes in lipid content and composition. The content of phospholipids and glucosylceramides in the SC is reduced, whereas the ceramide and free fatty acid contents are elevated. The major lipid classes in the SC are ceramides (CER, about 45%), free fatty acids (FFA, about 15%) and cholesterol (CHOL, about 25%). They are present in a roughly 1:1:1 molar ratio (Wertz and Norlén, 2003). Smaller amounts of cholesterol sulfate (2–5%) and cholesterol esters are also present. The lipid content varies between individuals and with anatomical site (Lampe et al., 1983). The most characteristic features for the SC lipid composition are: (1) extensive compositional heterogeneity with broad chain length distributions (mostly 20–32 carbon atoms (C); peaking at 24C) in the ceramide fatty acid and free fatty acid fractions, (2) an almost complete dominance of saturated very long hydrocarbon chains (C20:0–C32:0) and (3) large relative amounts of cholesterol (about 30 mol%) (Norlén, 2015). In addition, ceramide head groups are very small and contain several functional groups that can form lateral hydrogen bonds with adjacent ceramide molecules and other lipids. The increased chain length and the small size of the head group of ceramides, and the saturated long-chain FFA result in a very densely packed structure. Intercellular lipids are, therefore, arranged in a crystalline sublattice and only a small proportion of lipids form a liquid phase. Lipids in a crystalline or gel phase are far less permeable to water than those in a liquid phase. All these factors favor the function of the SC intercellular lipids as a barrier (Downing and Stewart, 2000; Lindberg and Forslind, 2000; Bouwstra et al., 2003). In addition, the bound lipids of the corneocyte lipid envelope are largely saturated lipids with a high melting point and function as a permeability barrier around each corneocyte and contribute to the formation and maintenance of the intercellular lipid lamellae (Downing and Stewart, 2000).

Regarding ceramides in human skin (HCER), at least eleven classes of ceramides, encompassing 342 individual ceramide species, have been identified in the human *stratum corneum*, and new ceramide species continue to be identified (Masukawa et al., 2006, 2008, 2009). Each ceramide molecule consists of a sphingoid moiety (sphingosine, phytosphingosine, 6-hydroxysphingosine or dihydrosphingosine) containing a polar head group and a hydrocarbon chain, as well as another hydrocarbon chain derived from a fatty acid or fatty acid ester moiety. Thus, HCER differ from each other by the head-group architecture (mainly sphingosine or phytosphingosne base linked to either a fatty acid, a α-hydroxy fatty acid or a ω-hydroxy fatty acid) and the hydrocarbon chain length. Increased level of sphingosine-based CERs at the expense of phytosphingosine-based CERs, as observed in the diseased skin, may contribute to the barrier function impairment (Uche et al., 2019). The ceramides containing a fatty acid ester moiety have an exceptionally long hydrocarbon chain, i.e. fatty acid ester-containing ceramides contain a markedly larger number (66–72) of carbon atoms compared to the typical ceramides containing a total of 38–54 carbon atoms (Masukawa et al. 2008). Further, as aforementioned, the polar head groups of ceramides form lateral hydrogen bonds and the hydrocarbon chains of ceramides are mostly saturated, which contributes to the rigid gel state of the extracellular lipids. The structure of some ceramides is represented in Figure 1.2.

HCER can be classified based on their polarity, with HCER 1 being the least polar. HCER1 (or acylceramide) and HCER4 have an exceptional molecular structure, in which a linoleic acid is linked to an ω-hydroxy fatty acid with a chain length of approximately 30–32 carbon atoms (Downing and Stewart, 2000; Bouwstra et al., 2003). It has been suggested that CER1 may serve as a molecular rivet to stabilize the multilamelar lipid array in the SC. Hence, the ω-hydroxyacyl chain would completely span one bilayer while the linoleate tail would insert into the adjacent layer (Schmidt, 1992; Wertz, 1992). Cholesterol has a role in the formation of lamellar organization of the SC lipids (Bouwstra et al., 1996). It enhances the formation of the highly dense orthorhombic lateral packing. Therefore, it is an indispensable component of the SC lipid matrix and is of fundamental importance for appropriate dense lipid organization and thus important for the skin barrier function (Mojumdar et al., 2015). In addition, cholesterol fluidizes the SC lipid bilayers at skin temperature (Zbytovska et al., 2009). Cholesterol sulfate has a role in maintaining the lamellar phase of lipids (Williams, 1984). It is thought to bond the adjacent lipid bilayers by forming bridges via divalent cations

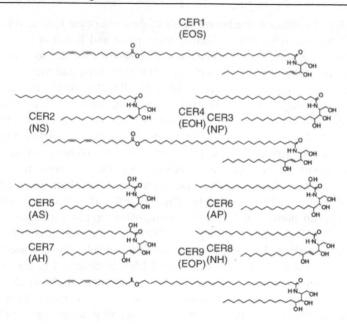

FIGURE 1.2 Molecular structure of ceramides (CER). CER in human stratum corneum. CER1, CER4 and CER9 have an ω-hydroxy acyl chain to which a linoleic acid is chemically linked (Bouwstra and Ponec, 2006).

(Wertz et al., 1987; Downing, 1992). In addition, cholesterol sulfate induces cohesion between adjacent corneocytes (Lampe et al., 1983).

The low permeability of the SC is not only due to the unique lipid composition, but rather to the unique structural organization of the lipid phase. The precise molecular organization of the SC lipids within the extracellular matrix remains a subject of intense investigation. There is a number of molecular models being proposed to elucidate SC lipid organization, and here are some of them presented.

Bouwstra et al. (2001) used small-angle X-ray diffraction to investigate the organization of the intercellular SC lipids. The results revealed that in untreated SC two lamellar phases are present, one with a periodicity of approximately 6.4 nm (short periodicity phase [SPP]) and the other with 13.4 nm (long periodicity phase [LPP]), together with a fluid phase (Figure 1.3). Since the 13 nm phase is always present in all species and is characteristic for the SC lipid phase behavior, this phase is probably important for the skin barrier function. They proposed a "sandwich model" with a repeating unit, which consists of three lipid layers: one narrow central lipid layer with fluid domains sandwiched between two adjacent broader

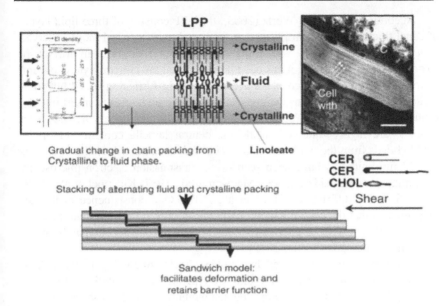

FIGURE 1.3 Model for molecular arrangement of the long periodicity phase (LPP). The presence of a broad-narrow-broad sequence in the repeating unit of the LPP (arrows) (left panel) is in agreement with the broad-narrow-broad pattern found in RuO4 fixed stratum corneum (right panel). CER1 plays an important role in dictating the broad-narrow-broad sequence. The fluid phase is located in the central narrow band. In adjacent regions the crystallinity is gradually increasing from the central layer. Bouwstra proposed a "sandwich model", which permits deformation while barrier function is retained (Bouwstra and Ponec, 2006).

layers with a crystalline structure. Ceramides are packed into a crystalline lattice within the broader phases. However, the long linoleate moieties in CER 1 and CER 4 protrude beyond the thickness of the crystalline phases into the space between the crystalline phases to form the narrow liquid phase with cholesterol. This liquid phase is proposed to be the main permeation pathway within the LPP (Bowstra et al., 2001). The lattice spacing within these three layers has been measured and the lipid packing was identified as orthorhombic (crystalline), hexagonal (gel-like) and liquid, corresponding to low, medium and high permeability, respectively (Bouwstra and Ponec, 2006). The change from orthorhombic to hexagonal packing in human SC, does not have an effect on the permeability. However, a perturbed lamellar organization revealed an increased skin permeability, indicating that a proper lamellar organization is more crucial for a competent barrier function than the presence of an orthorhombic lateral packing (Groen et al., 2011).

According to Hill and Wertz (2003), the LPP consists of three lipid layers of equal thickness. They proposed that the broad-narrow-broad motif observed under electron microscopy with ruthenium tetroxide fixation is an artifact. In these trilamellar structures, it has been proposed that the ω-hydroxyacyl portion of the acyl ceramide, which plays a central role in formation of 13 nm trilamellar lipid structures, spans the outer layers, while the linoleates insert into the central lamella (Hill and Wertz, 2003). With this arrangement, the outer two lamellae are highly saturated, while the central lamella contains all of the double bonds from the linoleate chains. This stabilizes the trilamellar structures into 13 nm units that have been seen using transmission electron microscopy with ruthenium tetroxide fixation (Madison et al., 1987; Kuempel et al., 1998) and with X-ray diffraction (Groen et al., 2010). One consequence of this arrangement is that the central lamella will reduce more ruthenium than the outer lamellae. This results in alternating broad-narrow-broad lucent bands in the electron micrographs (Wertz, 2015).

Another model is proposed by Norlén (2001). According to the author, compositional features of the SC lipids are typically those stabilizing lipid gel-phases. Therefore, it has been proposed that the horny layer lipid structure exists as a single and coherent gel phase (Norlén, 2001). The same group investigated the molecular organization of SC lipids *in situ* with the aid of a novel experimental approach: high-resolution cryo-electron microscopy of vitreous tissue section (CEMOVIS) and found that the lipid material is organized in the form of stacked bilayers of fully extended ceramides with cholesterol molecules associated with the ceramide sphingoid moiety. The viscous gel-like behavior of the lipid structure has been demonstrated by its remarkable malleability *in situ* (Iwai et al., 2012). This organization of lipids is responsible for the low permeability of the skin barrier and its robustness (Norlén, 2015).

1.3 DERMAL AND TRANSDERMAL DRUG DELIVERY

1.3.1 Therapeutic Target Sites in Dermal and Transdermal Delivery

During the development of drug formulations for the application onto the skin, it is important to distinguish between topical, regional and systemic drug delivery, as each drug delivery has its specificities and requirements. When

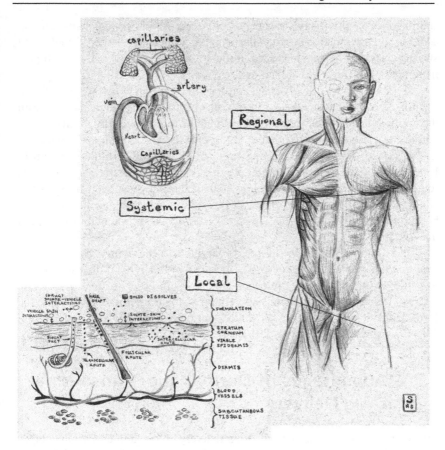

FIGURE 1.4   Targets in dermal and transdermal drug delivery (Predic Atkinson et al., 2015).

applied onto the skin, drugs should follow a route to one of the following target sites (Figure1.4):

1. local tissues immediately beneath the application site,
2. deep regions in the skin remote from the application site
3. systemic circulation (Flynn and Weiner, 1991).

Topical delivery can be defined as the application of a drug-containing formulation to the skin to directly treat cutaneous disorders or the cutaneous manifestations of a general disease. Topically delivered drugs should have their pharmacological or other effects confined to the surface of the skin or within the skin. Formulations designed to target the skin surface include barrier products, antimycotics, antipsoriatics, cosmetics, sunscreens, insect repellents, etc. In addition to these, topical formulations can target appendages (hair follicles and sweat pores) and include anti-acne products, antiperspirants, hair growth promoters and anti-infectives (Flynn and Weiner, 1991).

Regional delivery involves the application of a drug to the skin in order to treat diseases or alleviate disease symptoms in tissues that lie deeper, beneath the application site. Pharmacological targets of this type of drug delivery are within the musculature, vasculature, joints and tissues beneath and around the site of application. When targeting regional sites, drug formulations aim to have a regionally selective effect. Regional drug concentrations upon this route of drug administration are higher than the ones achieved by systemic administration (Flynn and Weiner, 1991; Benson and Watkinson, 2012). For both topical and regional drug delivery, systemic absorption is unwanted, but unavoidable.

In *transdermal delivery*, drugs are applied to the skin with the aim of reaching the systemic circulation. The purpose of this type of drug delivery is to achieve a therapeutically relevant drug level in order to treat a systemic disease. Hence, the percutaneous absorption of the drug is essential, while the local deposition of the drug is unwanted, but unavoidable (Flynn and Weiner, 1991; Benson and Watkinson, 2012).

1.3.2 Advantages of Dermal and Transdermal Drug Delivery

Transdermal, as well as dermal drug delivery, have numerous advantages compared to other conventional routes (Marwah et al., 2016; Paudel et al., 2010; Prausnitz and Langer, 2008):

1. Transdermal drug delivery systems (TDDS) avoid hepatic first-pass, which allows for lower doses of drugs to be administered, and that means these methods are safer for patients with liver diseases, resulting in the reduction of adverse effects;
2. Topical drug delivery systems are non-invasive, avoid hepatic first-pass as well as the gastrointestinal tract and problems associated with this drug application route, increase patient compliance and can be self-administered.
3. TDDS are an acceptable, pain-free, non-invasive form of self-administration for patients which ensures easy patient compliance and quick ending of the therapy if necessary;

4. Specially designed topical delivery systems (like liposomes) may also form drug "depots" in the skin with sustained drug release.
5. Topical drug delivery systems allow the drug to be directly applied to the skin and delivered to the site of disease in the skin.
6. TDDS avoid the gastrointestinal tract and so bypasses problems, such as drastic pH changes, the deleterious presence of food enzymes, variable transit times, rapidly fluctuating drug plasma concentrations;
7. TDDS act as a "depot" controlling the rate of drug input over a prolonged period of time and ensuring constant plasma levels even for drugs with short half lives. In the case of drugs with a narrow therapeutic margin, when applied onto the skin in TDDS, their undesirable side effects are reduced, particularly the effects associated with pulsed peak plasma levels. Furthermore, the dose interval can be reduced.

Due to these advantages there are numerous studies investigating dermal as well as transdermal drug delivery systems. However, the market is still limited to a narrow range of drugs, especially when TDD should be achieved (see Table 1.1). The problems that topical/transdermal drug delivery systems encounter are the low permeability of the SC, which limits the number of drugs available, and the potential interaction of drugs with the skin causing irritation and sensitization. The small number of drug candidates is due to the fact that only a few drug molecules have skin permeability coefficients sufficiently high to achieve clinically active plasma levels, i.e. for a successful TDD, drugs must have molecular weight (MW) less than 500 Daltons, be moderately lipohilic, have melting point <250°C and require doses of milligrams per day or less (daily systemic dose <20 mg, high potency drugs) (Benson, 2005; Prausnitz and Langer, 2008; Al Hanbali et al., 2019). Currently, the market for transdermal patches comprises patches with a few low molecular weight drugs: scopolamine for motion sickness, clonidine and nitroglycerin for cardiovascular disease, fentanyl for chronic pain, nicotine to aid smoking cessation, oestradiol (alone or in combination with levonorgestrel or norethisterone) for hormone replacement and testosterone for hypogonadism, etc. (see Table 1.1).

Particular challenges for TDD are hydrophilic drugs, peptides and macromolecules, including DNA and small-interfering RNA for gene therapy, and especially vaccines (Prausnitz and Langer, 2008). The vaccine delivery via the skin is most attractive among other mentioned candidates, as it targets in the skin the potent epidermal Langerhans and dermal dendritic cells, that may generate a strong immune response at much lower doses than deeper injection (Zheng et al., 2018).

TABLE 1.1 List of transdermal products on the market

	GENERIC DRUG	INDICATION	PRODUCT	MANUFACTURER
1	Scopolamine	Motion sickness	Transderm Scop®	Novartis
2	Nitroglycerin	Angina pectoris	Minitran®; Nitrol®; Transderm-Nitro®; Nitro-Dur®	3M; Rorer; Novartis; Key Pharms
3	Clonidine	Hypertension	Catapres-TTS®	Boehringer Ingelheim
4	Estradiol	Postmenopausal related symptoms	Estraderm®; Climara®	Novartis; Bayer Healthcare
5	Nicotine	Smoking cessation	Nicoderm CQ®; Habitrol®	Sanofi Aventis; Novartis
6	Testosteron	Hypogonadism	Androderm®; Testoderm®	Watson Labs; Alza
7	Fentanyl	Analgesia	Duragesic®	Janssen Pharmaceuticals
8	Estradiol and levonorgestrel	Postmenopausal related symptoms	Climara Pro™	Bayer Healthcare
9	Estradiol and norethindrone	Postmenopausal related symptoms	Combipatch®	Novartis
10	Ethinyl estradiol and norelgestromin	Contraception	Ortho Evra®	Janssen Pharmaceuticals
11	Buprenorphine	Analgesia	Bu Trans®	Purdue Pharma L.P.
12	Rivastigmine	Dementia associated with Alzheimer's and Parkinson's disease	Exelon®	Novartis
13	Oxybutynin	Overactive bladder	Oxytrol®; Kentera®	Watson Labs; Orion Pharma

(Continued)

TABLE 1.1 *(Continued)*

14	Oxybutynin chloride	Overactive bladder	Gelnique®	Watson Labs;
15	Rotigotine	Parkinson's disease	Neupro®	UCB Inc
16	Granisetron	Nausea, vomiting	Sancuso®	Prostrakan Inc
17	Methylphenidate	*Attention deficit hyperactivity disorder*	Daytrana;	Noven Pharms Inc
18	Selegiline	Depression	Emsam®	Somerset
19	Lidocaine	Postherpetic neuralgia pain relief	Lidoderm®	Teikoku Phar;
20	Lidocaine and tetracaine	Local dermal analgesia	Synera®	Zars Pharm
21	Capsaicin	Postherpetic neuralgia pain relief	Qutenza®	NeurogesX
22	Diclofenac epolamine	Topical pain relief	Flector®	Inst Biochem
23	Diclofenac sodium	Topical pain relief in osteoarthritis	Voltaren®	Novartis

Source: Predic Atkinson et al., 2015

As to TDDS, Prausnitz and Langer (2008) proposed categorizing them into three generations of development. Drugs in the 1st generation of TDDS have low MW, are lipophillic, achieve efficacy at low doses and generally do not require penetration enhancement. The 2nd generation of TDDS utilize penetration enhancement methods, such as: chemical enhancers, iontophoresis and non-cavitational ultrasound, but have been limited to the delivery of small MW molecules. The 3rd generation of TDDS delivers macromolecules to the SC with the help of novel chemical enhancers, electroporation, cavitational ultrasound, microneedles, thermal ablation and microdermabrasion.

To summarize, there is an emergency for skin penetration enhancement methods able to increase percutaneous drug penetration on one hand (see Section 1.6), while decreasing skin irritation on the other hand. This would open the dermal/transdermal market for hydrophilic compounds, macromolecules and conventional drugs for new therapeutic applications (Paudel et al., 2010, Predic Atkinson et al., 2015; Dragicevic and Maibach, 2015, 2016).

1.4 DRUG TRANSPORT ROUTES THROUGH THE SKIN

At the skin surface, a molecule has three possible routes to reach the viable tissue: (1) across the transcellular route, (2) across the intercellular route, and (1) via the appendages (Figure 1.5).

The transcellular route leads directly across the SC, involving the drug transport through keratinocytes and intercellular lipid lamellae. Hence, a molecule crossing SC via this route faces numerous repeating hurdles. The nature of the permeant and the partitioning coefficient will influence the importance of this route. Hydrophilic molecules may prefer the transcellular route at a pseudo-steady state. However, lipid bilayers are the rate-limiting barrier for permeation via this route (Williams, 2003; Benson and Watkinson, 2012).

The intercellular route is through the lipid bilayers, which comprise around 1% of the SC diffusional area, yet provide the only continuous phase within the membrane. It is generally accepted that, except for some

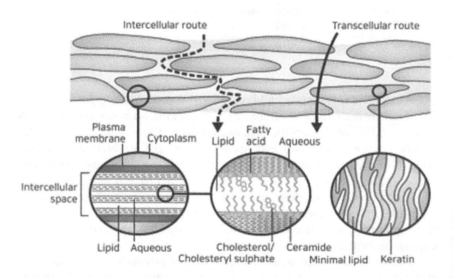

FIGURE 1.5 Penetration routes through SC: (1) intercellular route (2) transcellular route. (Barry, 2001).

specialized cases (e.g. highly hydrophilic substances), the intercellular lipid route is the principal pathway by which most small, uncharged molecules traverse the SC (Loth, 1992; Abraham et al., 1995; Roberts et al., 1996; Van Kuijk-Meuwissen et al., 1998; Benson and Watkinson, 2012) and many methods for enhancing the drug penetration disrupt or bypass the intercellular lipid bilayers of the SC (Barry, 2006). According to the domain mosaic model of the skin barrier (Forslind, 1994) the structural organization of the lipids of the SC has two phases: (1) lipids in crystalline/gel state surrounded by (2) lipids that form more fluid (liquid) crystalline domains. This second, more fluid lipid domains provide the pathway by which permeants traverse the SC.

The transappendageal transport (shunt route transport) involves the transport through the pilosebaceous units (hair follicles with sebaceous glands) and sweat ducts. Hair follicles are the most important appendage in terms of surface area (Schaefer and Redelmeier, 1996). Because of the low fractional appendageal area (about 0.1%) (Scheuplein, 1967), except for ions and highly polar molecules that struggle to cross intact stratum corneum, it was believed that this pathway usually adds little to steady-state drug flux (Scheuplein, 1967; Redelmeier and Kitson 1999; Agarwal et al., 2000). In recent years the follicular route has attracted considerable attention as an important penetration pathway, since it was realized that hair follicles, despite occupying only a small area of the total skin surface, represent invaginations extending deep into the dermis, which significantly increases their actual surface area available for penetration (Knorr et al., 2009), and they are surrounded by a dense network of blood capillaries (Vogt and Blume-Peytavi, 2003; Vogt et al., 2005). However, follicular penetration is a complex process, where it has to be distinguished between the "intrafollicular" penetration into the hair follicle (first step) and the "transfollicular" penetration into the living tissue surrounding the hair follicle (Figure 1.6), which cannot be observed for every applied substance, yet (Patzelt and Lademann, 2015).

The physicochemical properties of topically administered drug-loaded particles, such as size, determine its follicular penetration depth (Patzelt et al., 2011), and whether or not it is able to penetrate transfollicularly. Drug delivery via the hair follicles provides additional features such as fast delivery into the systemic circulation if transfollicular penetration is applicable (Otberg et al., 2008), as well as long-term intrafollicular storage for topically applied drugs if transfollicular penetration cannot be realized (Lademann et al., 2006, 2008, 2011). This long-term storage effect could be used for therapeutic purposes as the application of drug-loaded particles

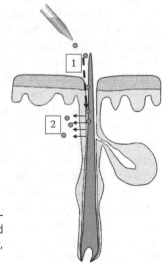

FIGURE 1.6   Follicular penetration pathway occurs in two steps: (1) intrafollicular penetration and (2) transfollicular penetration (Patzelt and Lademann, 2015).

with retarded drug release could diminish the application frequency and, thus, increase the compliance of patients and the therapeutic outcome (Patzelt and Lademann, 2015). Further, appendages may function as shunts, which may be important at short times prior to steady-state diffusion (Barry, 2006). It has been shown that the follicular route may be especially important for the hydrophilic molecules (Otberg et al., 2008), molecules with high molecular weight (Dokka et al., 2005) and for different particulate-based drug delivery systems, which show a high tendency to aggregate in the hair follicle openings (Essa et al., 2002; Alvarez-Roman et al., 2004; Shim et al., 2004; Toll et al., 2004; Ossadnik et al., 2006; Baroli et al., 2007; Rouse et al., 2007). It has been shown that especially nanoparticles were able to permeate the skin passively through the hair follicle and improve drug penetration into the hair follicle (Lademann et al., 2007; Rancan et al., 2009; Toll et al., 2004). Lademann et al. (2007) found *in vitro* in porcine skin a preferential deposition of poly(d,l-lactic-co-glycolic acid) (PLGA) nanoparticles of 320 nm in diameter in hair follicles, demonstrating a size dependency. The fluorescent dye encapsulated in these nanoparticles penetrated significantly deeper into the hair follicles than the same free dye. Rancan et al. (2009) reported deposition of polylactic nanoparticles of 228 and 365 nm in diameter in 50% of the available vellus hair follicles. Wang et al. (2008) demonstrated *in vitro* in human skin deposition of PLGA nanoparticles around hair follicles and sebaceous glands. It has been demonstrated that particles of approximately 400–700 nm showed the deepest penetration into the hair follicles, where they were stored longer than in the

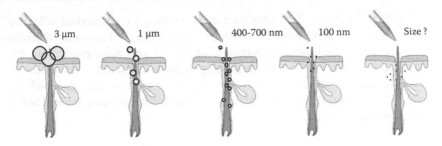

FIGURE 1.7   Particle size-dependent penetration depth of the particles. Particles of 400–700 nm in diameter penetrate significantly deeper into the hair follicles than larger or smaller particles (Patzelt and Lademann, 2015).

SC, whereas larger and smaller particles reached significantly lower penetration depths (Patzelt et al. 2011) or remained even on the skin surface in the case of very large particles (Schaefer and Lademann 2001; Toll et al. 2004). Thus, the penetration depth of the particles can be influenced by their size (Figure 1.7) resulting in the possibility of a differentiated targeting of specific follicular structures. Further, in contrast to free drugs (rhodamine B (Rh B) and fluorescein isothiocyanate [FITC], which showed a negligible skin penetration and localization in hair follicles, the drug-loaded nanoparticles were preferentially deposited in hair follicles (Küchler et al., 2009; Alvarez-Roman et al., 2004).

Liposomes have been also used to target the hair follicle (Li et al., 1992, 1993a,b; Lieb et al., 1992; Li and Hoffman 1997; Hoffman, 1998; Ciotti and Weiner 2002; Jung et al., 2006), which is discussed in Chapter 2. It has been shown that molecules can penetrate through the hair follicle into the blood (Otberg et al., 2008; Blume-Peytavi et al., 2010; Grice et al., 2010). In addition, the hair follicles contain multiple associated target structures, such as immune cells (like antigen-presenting cells, mast cells and others), stem cells and melanocytes, sebaceous glands and perifollicular blood vessels, which are accessible for innovative therapeutic approaches (Vogt et al., 2005; Knorr et al., 2009). Therefore, they are a promising target, especially for sebaceous glands (Bernard et al., 1997; Münster et al., 2005), as well as for transcutaneous (i.e. transfollicular) gene therapy and immunization, which can be achieved by the use of elastic vesicles (Hoffman, 1998, 2016; Christoph et al., 2000; Gupta et al., 2001; Cotsarelis, 2002; Gupta et al., 2005a,b; Vogt et al., 2006, 2008). Targeting the hair follicle stem cells by gene transfer via nanocarriers represents a promising option for the treatment of genetic hair diseases and skin diseases (Ohyama and Vogel, 2003; Sugiyama-Nakagiri et al., 2006). Frum et al. (2008) showed that formulation variables (pH, viscosity and addition of penetration enhancers) may have a marked influence on the follicular permeation of topically applied drugs. Thus, the follicular route is gaining increasing importance for dermal and transdermal drug delivery and smart nanocarrier-based drug delivery systems, such as nanoparticles and novel elastic liposomes represent a promising approach to increase the percutaneous drug absorption via this permeation route (Patzelt and Lademann, 2015, 2020).

1.5 FACTORS AFFECTING DRUG PERMEATION RATE THROUGH THE SKIN

Factors affecting the drug permeation rate through the SC can be considered using the equation (Eq. (1.1)) for steady state flux (Barry, 1991):

$$\frac{dm}{dt} = \frac{DC_0P}{h} \tag{1.1}$$

where dm/dt is the steady state flux, presenting the cumulative mass of the diffusant, m, passing per unit area through the membrane, C_0 is the constant donor drug concentration, P is the partition coefficient of a solute between membrane and bathing solution, D is the diffusion coefficient and h is the membrane thickness. From Eq. (1.1), the ideal properties for a molecule in order to penetrate SC well, would be the following (Barry, 2001; Benson, 2005):

- Low molecular weight, preferably less than 600 Da, when D tends to be high.
- Adequate solubility in oil and water in order to achieve a high membrane concentration gradient, which is the driving force for diffusion (C_0 is large).
- High, but balanced P (log P octanol/water of 1 to 3) since a too high coefficient may inhibit clearance from viable tissues. Drugs should have adequate solubility within lipid domains of the SC (to permit diffusion through this domain), whilst still having a sufficiently hydrophilic nature to allow partitioning into the viable epidermis.
- Low melting point, which correlates with good solubility as predicted by the ideal solubility theory.

When a drug possesses the aforementioned ideal physicochemical properties (as in the case of nicotine and nitroglycerin), transdermal delivery is feasible. If the drug does not match these ideal characteristics, manipulation of the drug or vehicle to enhance diffusion is necessary, and/or penetration enhancement techniques are to be used.

1.6 PENETRATION ENHANCEMENT TECHNIQUES-CLASSIFICATION

Since percutaneous absorption is pivotal to the effectiveness of both dermal and transdermal systems, significant efforts have been devoted to developing strategies to overcome the impermeability of the intact human skin. There are many methods for circumventing the SC (Figure 1.8), thereby enhancing the drug delivery into/through the skin. They can be classified in different ways, e.g. into chemical (such as chemical penetration enhancers, use of prodrugs, supersaturation, complexes, ion pairs, vesicles and other nanocarriers, etc.) and physical penetration enhancement methods (such as iontophoresis, electroporation, ultrasound, microneedles) (Williams and Barry, 2004; Benson, 2005; Prausnitz and Langer, 2008; Predic Atkinson et al., 2015; Dragicevic and Maibach, 2015a,b, 2016, 2017).

Among different penetration enhancement methods, in this chapter chemical penetration enhancers will be discussed in brief, as they may be constituents of novel elastic vesicles (e.g. terpenes as ingredients in invasomes, ethanol in ethosomes, surfactants in penetration enhancer - containing vesicles, etc.)

1.6.1 Chemical Penetration Enhancers

Chemical penetration enhancers (also known as accelerants or sorption promoters, CPEs or PEs) currently represent the most widely studied approach to enhance dermal/transdermal delivery of drugs (Williams and Barry, 2004; Ahad et al., 2009; Rizwan et al., 2009; Dragicevic and Maibach, 2016). CPEs are defined as agents that partition into, and interact with the SC constituents to induce a temporary, reversible increase in skin permeability. These substances temporarily reduce skin resistance and thereby enhance drug flux (Barry, 2001).

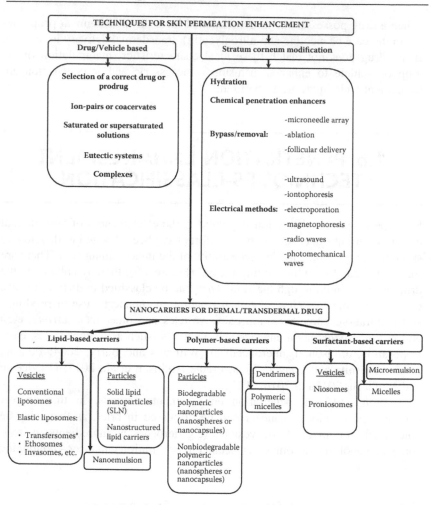

FIGURE 1.8   Penetration enhancement methods.

Different groups of structurally related chemical compounds are used as penetration enhancers: surfactants, essential oils, terpenes and their derivatives, fatty acids, esters, ethers, Azone® and its derivatives, Transcutol®, transkarbams, amides, sulphoxides and their analogs, pyrrolidones, etc. (Babu and Chen, 2015; Dragicevic and Maibach, 2016; Heard, 2015; Jampilek, 2015; Javazadeh et al., 2015; Ramezanli et al., 2015). Besides being potent penetration enhancers, CPEs show also limitations as they often irritate the skin and do not achieve the desired skin disruption (they have often low efficacy at therapeutical levels). In attempts to solve these problems, researchers have tried synthesizing novel chemical penetration

TABLE 1.2   Modes of action of chemical penetration enhancers

MECHANISM	EFFECT ON SKIN PERMEABILITY	PE ACTING VIA THIS MECHANISM
Disruption of the intercellular bilayer lipid structure (Lipid modification) Fluidization of SC lipids Lipid extraction Polar head group alteration	D increases	Azone®, terpenes, fatty acids, dimethyl sulfoxide (DMSO), and alcohols
Interaction with intracellular proteins of the SC (Protein modification) and with corneocytes Opening up the dense keratin structure and binding with keratin filaments→ disruption of the order within corneocytes Interaction with SC desmosomes Corneocytes alteration	D increases	Ionic surfactants, decylmethylsulphoxide and DMSO, urea
Improvement of drug, coenhancer or cosolvent partitioning into the SC (Partitioning promotion) PE changes *stratum corneum* solubility properties closer to that of the permeant	Increase of drug partitioning into the SC and solubility within the SC	Ethanol, propylene glycol, diethylene glycol monoethyl ether (Transcutol®), N-methyl pyrrolidone
"Drag effect"- solvent permeating the skin carries the permeant with it	Increase of partitioning	Ethanol, propylene glycol

enhancers, with optimal enhancer features (Akimoto and Nagase, 2003), or using two or more penetration enhancers together, because of their synergistic effect in augmenting the penetration of drugs into/through skin (Furuishi et al., 2010).

Barry and coworkers (Barry, 1991; Williams and Barry, 1991) introduced the lipid-protein-partitioning (LPP) theory to categorize penetration enhancers and to describe the mechanism by which penetration enhancers affect skin permeability. According to this theory and results of numerious studies (Cornwell et al., 1994a, 1996; Williams and Barry, 2004; Benson, 2005; Shah et al., 2008; Hatta et al., 2010, Chen et al., 2016), enhancers act by one or more of the three direct modes of action, as well as by the indirect mode ("drag effect") (Table 1.2.).

1.7 CONCLUSION

In the last few decades, the research focus of dermal and transdermal drug delivery has been on improving skin permeability through the development of new penetration enhancement methods which would enhance the percutaneous drug penetration. Chemical enhancement methods, such as chemical penetration enhancers and especially different vesicles i.e. novel vesicles, being deformable/elastic due to the presence of chemical penetration enhancers in their composition (e.g. invasomes, transfersomes, ethosomes, penetration enhancer-containing vesicles (PEV)), have been extensively studied in the last decades, as they have shown to be promising in enhancing drug delivery into/through the skin. The phospholipid vesicles, such as invasomes, which are the main topic of this book, have, however, a crucial advantage over chemical penetration enhancers, as they are non-harmful, non-irritating, non-immunogenic, and without allergic potential.

A further aim of dermal and especially transdermal drug delivery systems is to extend the list of products on the market, both in terms of diversity of drug compounds and range of indications (diseases) treated. One way forward would be including more macromolecular drug formulations, especially vaccines, and the recent penetration enhancement methods' development is promising to push these boundaries.

REFERENCES

Abdulmajed, K., Heard, C.M., 2008. Topical delivery of retinyl ascorbate. 3. Influence of follicle sealing and skin stretching. *Skin Pharm. Physiol.* 21(1), 46–49.

Abraham, M.H., Chanda, H.S., Mitchell, R.C., 1995. The factors that influence skin penetration of solutes. *J. Pharm. Pharmacol.* 47, 8–16.

Agarwal, R., Katare, O.P., Vyas, S.P., 2000 Mar. The pilosebaceous unit: a pivotal route for topical drug delivery. *Methods Find Exp. Clin. Pharmacol.* 22(2), 129–133.

Ahad, A., Aqil, M., Kohli, K., Chaudhary, H., Sultana, Y., Mujeeb, M., et al., 2009 Jul. Chemical penetration enhancers: a patent review. *Expert Opin. Ther. Pat.* 19(7), 969–988.

Akimoto, T., Nagase, Y., 2003 Mar 7. Novel transdermal drug penetration enhancer: synthesis and enhancing effect of alkyldisiloxane compounds containing glucopyranosyl group. *J. Control Release.* 88(2), 243–252.

Al Hanbali, O.A., Khan, H.M.S., Sarfraz M., Arafat M., Ijaz S., Hameed, A. 2019 Jun 1. Transdermal patches: Design and current approaches to painless drug delivery. *Acta Pharm.* 69(2), 197–215.

Alvarez-Roman, R., Naik, A., Kalia, Y.N., Guy, R.H., Fessi, H., 2004. Skin penetration and distribution of polymeric nanoparticles. *J. Control. Release.* 99, 53–62.

Andrews, S.N., Jeong, E., Prausnitz, M.R., 2013 Apr. Transdermal Delivery of Molecules is Limited by Full Epidermis, Not Just Stratum Corneum. *Pharm. Res.* 30(4), 1099–1109.

Babu, R.J., Chen, L., 2015. Pyrrolidones as Penetration Enhancers. In: Dragicevic, N., Maibach, H. (eds) *Percutaneous Penetration Enhancers Chemical Methods in Penetration Enhancement.* Springer, Berlin, Heidelberg.

Baroli, B., Ennas, M.G., Loffredo, F., Isola, M., Pinna, R., Lopez-Quintela, M.A., 2007. Penetration of metallic nanoparticles in human full-thickness skin. *J. Invest. Dermatol.* 127, 1701–1712.

Barry, B.W., 1991. Lipid–protein-partititioning theory of skin penetration enhancement, *J. Control. Release.* 15, 237–248.

Barry, B.W., 2001. Novel mechanisms and devices to enable successful transdermal drug delivery. *Eur. J. Pharm. Sci.* 14(2), 101–114.

Barry, B.W., 2006. Penetration Enhancer Classification. In: Smith, E.W., Maibach, H.I. (eds) *Percutaneous Penetration Enhancers.* CRC Press, Taylor & Francis Group, LLC, Boca Raton, FL, pp. 3–15.

Benson, H.A.E., 2005 Jan. Transdermal drug delivery: penetration enhancement techniques. *Curr Drug Deliv.* 2(1), 23–33.

Benson, H.A.E., Watkinson, A.C., 2012. *Transdermal and Topical Drug Delivery: Principles and Practice.* Wiley, Hoboken, N.J.

Bernard, E., Dubois, J.L., Wepierre, J., 1997. Importance of sebaceous glands in cutaneous penetration of an antiandrogen: target effect of liposomes. *J. Pharm. Sci.* 86, 573–578.

Blume-Peytavi, U., Massoudy, L., Patzelt, A., Lademann, J., Dietz, E., Rasulev, U., Garcia Bartels, N., 2010. Follicular and percutaneous penetration pathways of topically applied minoxidil foam. *Eur. J. Pharm. Biopharm.* 76, 450–453.

Bouwstra, J.A., Ponec, M., 2006 Dec. The skin barrier in healthy and diseased state. *Biochim. Biophys. Acta.* 1758(12), 2080–2095.

Bouwstra, J.A., Honeywell-Nguyen, P.L., Gooris G.S., Ponec, M., 2003. Structure of the skin barrier and its modulation by vesicular formulations. *Progress in Lipid Res.* 42, 1–36.

Bouwstra, J., Pilgram, G., Gooris, G., Koerten, H., Ponec, M., 2001. New aspects of the skin barrier organization. *Skin Pharmacol. Appl. Skin Physiol.* 14 Suppl 1, 52–62.

Bouwstra, J.A., Gooris, G.S., Cheng, K., Weerheim, A., Bras, W., Ponec, M., 1996 Phase behavior of isolated skin lipids. *J. Lipid Res.* 37, 999–1011

Chen, J., Jiang, Q.D., Chai, Y.P., Zhang, H., Peng, P., Yang, X.X., 2016 Dec 11. Natural Terpenes as Penetration Enhancers for Transdermal Drug Delivery. *Molecules* 21(12), 1709.

Christoph, T., Müller-Röver, S., Audring, H., Tobin, D.J., Hermes, B., Cotsarelis, G., Rückert, R., Paus, R., 2000. The human hair follicle immune system: cellular composition and immune privilege. *Br. J. Dermatol.* 142, 862–873.

Ciotti, S.N., Weiner, N., 2002 May. Follicular liposomal delivery systems. *J. Liposome. Res.* 12(1-2), 143–148.

Cornwell, P.A., Barry, B.W., Stoddart, C.P., Bouwstra, J.A., 1994. Wide-angle X-ray diffraction of human stratum corneum: effects of hydration and terpene enhancer treatment. *J. Pharm. Pharmacol.* 46, 938–950.

Cornwell, P.A., Barry, B.W., Bouwstra, J.A., Gooris, G.S., 1996. Modes of action of terpene penetration enhancers in human skin; differential scanning calorimetry, small-angle X-ray diffraction and enhancer uptake studies. *Int. J. Pharm.* 127, 9–26.

Cotsarelis, G., 2002. Les follicules pilaires comme cibles de la thérapie génique [The hair follicle as a target for gene therapy]. *Ann. Dermatol. Venereol.*, 129(5 Pt 2), 841–844. French. PMID: 12223969.

Dokka, S., Cooper, S.R., Kelly, S., Hardee, G.E., Karras, J.G., 2005. Dermal delivery of topically applied oligonucleotides via follicular transport in mouse skin. *J. Invest. Dermatol.* 124, 971–975.

Downing, D.T., 1992. Lipid and protein structures in the permeability barrier of mammalian epidermis. *J. Lipid Res.* 33, 301–313.

Downing, D.T., Stewart, M.E., 2000. Epidermal Composition. In: Loden, M., Maibach, H.I. (eds) *Dry Skin and Moisturizers, Chemistry and Function*, Boca Raton, London, New York, pp. 13–26.

Downing, D.T., Lazo, N.D., 2000. Lipid and Protein Structures in the Permeability Barrier. In: Loden, M., Maibach, H.I. (eds) *Dry Skin and Moisturizers, Chemistry and Function*. Boca Raton, London, New York, pp. 39–44.

Dragicevic, N., Atkinson, J.P., Maibach, H.I., 2015. Chemical Penetration Enhancers: Classification and Mode of Action. In: Dragicevic N., Maibach H. (eds) *Percutaneous Penetration Enhancers, Chemical Methods in Penetration Enhancement, Modification of the Stratum corneum*. Springer, Berlin, Heidelberg, 93–108.

Dragicevic, N., Maibach, H. (eds.), 2015b. *Percutaneous Penetration Enhancers, Chemical Methods in Penetration Enhancement, Modification of the stratum corneum*. Springer, Berlin, Heidelberg.

Dragicevic, N., Maibach, H. (eds.), 2016. Percutaneous Penetration Enhancers, Chemical Methods in Penetration Enhancement. *Nanocarriers*, Springer, Berlin, Heidelberg.

Dragicevic, N., I. Maibach, H. (eds.), 2017. *Percutaneous Penetration Enhancers Physical Methods in Penetration Enhancement*. Springer, Berlin, Heidelberg.

El Maghraby, G.M., Williams, A.C., 2009 Feb. Vesicular systems for delivering conventional small organic molecules and larger macromolecules to and through human skin. *Expert Opin. Drug Deliv.* 6(2), 149–163.

Elias, P.M., 1983. Epidermal lipids, barrier function, and desquamation. *J Invest Dermatol.* 80 Suppl, 44s–49ss.

Essa, E.A., Bonner, M.C., Barry, B.W., 2002. Human skin sandwich for assessing shunt route penetration during passive and iontophoretic drug and liposome delivery. *J. Pharm. Pharmacol.* 54, 1481–1490.

Flynn, G.L., Weiner, N.D., 1991. Topical and Transdermal delivery-provinces of realism. In: Teubner, G.R., Teubner, A. (eds) *Dermal and Transdermal Delivery*. Wissenschaftliche Verlagsgesellschaft GmbH, Stuttgart, 33–64.

Forslind, B., 1994 Jan. A domain mosaic model of the skin barrier. *Acta Derm. Venereol.* 74(1), 1–6.

Frum, Y., Eccleston, G.M., Meidan, V.M., 2008. Factors influencing hydrocortisone permeation into human hair follicles: use of the skin sandwich system. *Int. J. Pharm.* 358, 144–150.

Furuishi, T., Fukami, T., Suzuki T., Takayama, K., Tomono, K., 2010. Synergistic effect of isopropyl myristate and glyceryl monocaprylate on the skin permeation of pentazocine. *Biol. Pharm. Bull.* 33(2), 294–300.

Grice, J.E., Ciotti, S., Weiner, N., Lockwood, P., Cross, S.E., Roberts, M.S., 2010. Relative uptake of minoxidil into appendages and stratum corneum and permeation through human skin in vitro. *J. Pharm. Sci.* 99, 712–718.

Groen, D., Gooris, G.S., Bouwstra, J.A., 2010. Model membranes prepared with ceramide EOS, cholesterol and free fatty acids form a unique lamellar phase. *Langmuir* 26, 4168–4175.

Groen, D., Poole, D.S., Gooris, G.S., Bouwstra, J.A., 2011 Jun. Is an orthorhombic lateral packing and a proper lamellar organization important for the skin barrier function? *Biochim. Biophys. Acta.* 1808(6), 1529–1537.

Gupta, S., Domashenko, A., Cotsarelis, G., 2001. The hair follicle as a target for gene therapy. *Eur. J. Dermatol.* 11, 353–356.

Gupta, P.N., Mishra, V., Singh, P., Rawat, A., Dubey, P., Mahor, S., Vyas, S.P., 2005a. Tetanus toxoid-loaded transfersomes for topical immunization. *J. Pharm. Pharmacol.* 57, 295–301.

Gupta, P.N., Mishra, V., Rawat, A., Dubey, P., Mahor, S., Jain, S., Chatterji, D.P., Vyas, S.P., 2005b. Non-invasive vaccine delivery in transfersomes, niosomes and liposomes: a comparative study. *Int. J. Pharm.* 293, 73–82.

Hatta, I., Nakazawa, H., Obata, Y., Ohta, N., Inoue, K., Yagi, N., 2010. Novel method to observe subtle structural modulation of stratum corneum on applying chemical agents. *Chem. Phys. Lipids* 163, 381–389.

Heard, C.M., 2015. Ethanol and Other Alcohols: Old Enhancers, Alternative Perspectives. In: Dragicevic N., Maibach H. (eds) *Percutaneous Penetration Enhancers Chemical Methods in Penetration Enhancement*. Springer, Berlin, Heidelberg.

Hill, J.R., Wertz, P.W., 2003. Molecular models of the intercellular lipid lamellae from epidermal stratum corneum. *Biochim. Biophys. Acta* 1616, 121–126.

Hoffman, R.M., 1998. Topical liposome targeting of dyes, melanins, genes, and proteins selectively to hair follicles. *J. Drug Target.* 5(2), 67–74.

Hoffman, R.M., 2016. Introduction to hair-follicle-associated pluripotent stem cells. *Methods Mol. Biol.* 1453, 1–5.

Iwai, I.H., H. den Hollander, L. Svensson, S. Öfverstedt, L.-G. Anwar, J. Brewer, J. Bloksgaard Mølgaard, M. Laloeuf, A. Nosek, D. Masich, S. Bagatolli, L. Skoglund, U. Norlén L., 2012. The human skin barrier is organized as stacked bilayers of fully-extended ceramides with cholesterol molecules associated with the ceramide sphingoid moiety. *J. Invest. Dermatol.* 132(9), 2215–2225.

Jampílek, J., 2015. Azone® and Its Analogues as Penetration Enhancers. In: Dragicevic N., Maibach H. (eds) *Percutaneous Penetration Enhancers Chemical Methods in Penetration Enhancement*. Springer, Berlin, Heidelberg, 69–105.

Javadzadeh, Y., Adibkia, K., Hamishekar, H., 2015. Transcutol® (Diethylene Glycol Monoethyl Ether): A Potential Penetration Enhancer. In: Dragicevic, N., Maibach, H. (eds) *Percutaneous Penetration Enhancers Chemical Methods in Penetration Enhancement*. Springer, Berlin, Heidelberg, 195–205.

Jung, S., Otberg, N., Thiede, G., Richter, H., Sterry, W., Panzner, S., Lademann, J., 2006. Innovative liposomes as a transfollicular drug delivery system: penetration into porcine hair follicles. *J. Invest. Dermatol.* 126, 1728–1732.

Knorr, F., Lademann, J., Patzelt, A., Sterry, W., Blume-Peytavi, U., Vogt, A., 2009. Follicular transport route – research progress and future perspectives. *Eur. J. Pharm. Biopharm.* 71, 173–180.

Küchler, S., Abdel-Mottaleb, M., Lamprecht, A., Radowski, M.R., Haag, R., Schäfer-Korting, M., 2009 Jul 30. Influence of nanocarrier type and size on skin delivery of hydrophilic agents. *Int. J. Pharm.* 377(1–2), 169–172.

Kuempel, D., Swartzendruber, D.C., Squier, C.A., Wertz, P.W., 1998. In vitro reconstruction of stratum corneum lipid lamellae. *Biochim. Biophys. Acta* 1372, 135–140.

Lademann, J., Richter, H., Schaefer, U.F., Blume-Peytavi, U., Teichmann, A., Otberg, N., Sterry, W., 2006. Hair follicles – a long-term reservoir for drug delivery. *Skin Pharmacol. Physiol.* 19, 232–236.

Lademann, J., Richter, H., Schanzer, S., Knorr, F., Meinke, M., Sterry, W., Patzelt A., 2011. Penetration and storage of particles in human skin: Perspectives and safety aspects. *Eur. J. Pharm. Biopharm.* 77, 465–468.

Lademann, J., Knorr, F., Richter, H., Blume-Peytavi, U., Vogt, A., Antoniou, C., Sterry, W., Patzelt A., 2008. Hair follicles – an efficient storage and penetration pathway for topically applied substances. *Skin Pharmacol. Physiol.* 21, 150–155.

Lademann, J., Richter, H., Teichmann, A., Otberg, N., Blume-Peytavi, U., Luengo, J., Weiss, B., Schaefer, U.F., Lehr, C.M., Wepf, R., Sterry, W., 2007. Nanoparticles – an efficient carrier for drug delivery into the hair follicles. *Eur. J. Pharm. Biopharm. (official journal of Arbeitsgemeinschaft fur Pharmazeutische Verfahrenstechnik eV)* 66 (2), 159–164.

Lampe, M.A., Williams, M.L., Elias, P.M., 1983. Human epidermal lipids: characterization and modulation during differentiation. *J. Lipid Res.* 24, 131–140.

Li, L., Hoffman, R.M., 1997. Topical liposome delivery of molecules to hair follicles in mice. *J. Derm. Sci.* 14, 101–108.

Li L., Hoffman, R.M., 1997 Feb. Topical liposome delivery of molecules to hair follicles in mice. *J. Dermatol. Sci.* 14(2), 101–108.

Li, L., Margolis, L.B., Lishko, L.V., 1992. Product-delivering liposomes specifically target entrapped melanin to hair follicles in histocultured intact skin. *In Vitro Cell. Dev. Biol.* 28A, 679–681.

Li, L., Lishko, L.V., Hoffman, R.M., 1993a. Liposomes can specifically target entrapped melanin to hair follicles in histocultured skin. *In Vitro Cell. Dev. Biol.* 29A, 192–194.

Li, L., Lishko, L.V., Hoffman, R.M., 1993b. Liposomes targeting high molecular weight DNA to hair follicles in histocultured skin: a model for gene therapy of the hair growth process. *In Vitro Cell. Dev. Biol.* 29A, 258–260.

Lieb, L.M., Ramachandran, C., Egbaria, K., Weiner, N., 1992. Topical delivery enhancement with multilamellar liposomes into pilosebaceous units. I. In vitro evaluation using fluorescent techniques with hamster ear model. *J. Invest. Dermatol.* 99, 108–113.

Lindberg, M., Forslind, B., 2000. The Skin as a Barrier. In: Loden, M., Maibach, H.I. (eds) *Dry Skin and Moisturizers, Chemistry and Function*, CRC Press/Taylor & Francis Group, Boca Raton, FL, pp. 27–37.

Loth, H., 1992. Percutaneous Absorption and Conventional Penetration Enhancers. In: Braun-Falco, O., Korting, H.C., Maibach, H.I. (eds) *Liposome Dermatics*, Springer-Verlag, Berlin, 3–10.

Madison, K.C., Swartzendruber, D.C., Wertz, P.W., Downing, D.T., 1987. Presence of intact intercellular lipid lamellae in the upper layers of the stratum corneum. *J. Invest. Dermatol.* 88, 714–718.

Marwah, H., Garg, T., Goyal, A.K., Rath, G., 2016. Permeation enhancer strategies in transdermal drug delivery. *Drug Deliv.* 23(2), 564–578.

Masukawa, Y., Tsujimura, H., Narita, H., 2006 Jul. Liquid chromatography-mass spectrometry for comprehensive profiling of ceramide molecules in human hair. *J. Lipid Res.* 47(7), 1559–1571.

Masukawa, Y., Narita, H., Sato, H., Naoe, A., Kondo, N., Sugai, Y., Oba, T., Homma, R., Ishikawa, J., Takagi, Y., Kitahara, T., 2009. Comprehensive quantification of ceramide species in human stratum corneum. *J. Lipid Res.* 50, 1708–1719

Masukawa, Y., Narita, H., Shimizu, E., Kondo, N., Sugai, Y., Oba, T., Homma, R., Ishikawa, J., Takagi, Y., Kitahara, T., Takema, Y., Kita, K., 2008. Characterization of overall ceramide species in human stratum corneum. *J. Lipid Res.* 49, 1466–1476

Mojumdar, E.H., Gooris, G.S., Bouwstra, J.A., 2015 Jun 7. Phase behavior of skin lipid mixtures: the effect of cholesterol on lipid organization. *Soft Matter.* 11(21), 4326–4336.

Münster, U., Nakamura, C., Haberland, A., Jores, K., Mehnert, W., Rummel, S., Schaller, M., Korting, H.C., Zouboulis, C., Blume-Peytavi, U., Schafer-Korting, M., 2005. RU 58841-myristate – prodrug development for topical treatment of acne and androgenetic alopecia. *Pharmazie* 60, 8–12.

Norlen, L., 2012. Skin Lipids. In: G.C.K. Roberts (ed) Springer *Encyclopedia of Biophysics*.

Norlén, L., 2001. Skin barrier structure and function: the single gel-phase model. *J. Invest. Dermatol.* 117(4), 830–836

Norlén, L., 2015. Molecular Structure and Function of the Skin Barrier. In: Dragicevic, N., Maibach, H. (eds) *Percutaneous Penetration Enhancers Chemical Methods in Penetration Enhancement*. Springer, Berlin, Heidelberg.

Ohyama, M., Vogel, J.C., 2003. Gene delivery to the hair follicle. *J. Invest. Dermatol. Symp. Proc.* 8, 204–206.

Ossadnik, M., Richter, H., Teichmann, A., Koch, S., Schafer, U., Wepf, R., Sterry, W., Lademann, J., 2006. Investigation of differences in follicular penetration of particle and nonparticle-containing emulsions by laser scanning microscopy. *Laser Phys.* 16, 747–750.

Otberg, N., Patzelt, A., Rasulev, U., Hagemeister, T., Linscheid, M., Sinkgraven, R., Sterry, W., Lademann, J., 2008. The role of hair follicles in the percutaneous absorption of caffeine. *Br. J. Clin. Pharmacol.* 65, 488–492.

Pandit, J., Aqil, M., Sultana, Y., 2015. Terpenes and Essential Oils as Skin Penetration Enhancers. In: Dragicevic, N., Maibach, H. (eds) *Percutaneous Penetration Enhancers Chemical Methods in Penetration Enhancement.* Springer, Berlin, Heidelberg.

Patzelt, A., Lademann, J., 2015. The Increasing Importance of the Hair Follicle Route in Dermal and Transdermal Drug Delivery. In: Dragicevic, N., Maibach, H. (eds) *Percutaneous Penetration Enhancers Chemical Methods in Penetration Enhancement.* Springer, Berlin, Heidelberg.

Patzelt, A., Richter, H., Knorr, F., Schäfer, U., Lehr, C.M., Dähne, L., Sterry, W., Lademann, J., 2011. Selective follicular targeting by modification of the particle sizes. *J. Control. Release* 150, 45–48.

Patzelt, A., Lademann, J., 2020. Recent advances in follicular drug delivery of nanoparticles. *Expert Opin. Drug Deliv.* 17(1), 49–60. doi: 10.1080/17425247. 2020.1700226. Epub 2019 Dec 12. PMID: 31829758.

Paudel, K.S., Milewski, M., Swadley, C.L., Brogden, N.K., Ghosh P., Stinchcomb, A.L., 2010 Jul. Challenges and opportunities in dermal/transdermal delivery. *Ther. Deliv.* 1(1), 109–131.

Prausnitz, M.R., Langer, R., 2008 Nov. Transdermal drug delivery. *Nat. Biotechnol.* 26(11), 1261–1268.

Predic Atkinson, P., Maibach, H.I., Dragicevic, N., 2015. Targets in Dermal and Transdermal Delivery and Classification of Penetration Enhancement Methods. In: Dragicevic, N., Maibach, H. (eds) *Percutaneous Penetration Enhancers Chemical Methods in Penetration Enhancement.* Springer, Berlin, Heidelberg.

Ramezanli, T., Tsai, P.C., Dorrani, M., Michniak-Kohn, B.B., 2015. Aromatic Iminosulfuranes, A Novel Class of Transdermal Penetration Enhancers. In: Dragicevic, N., Maibach, H. (eds) *Percutaneous Penetration Enhancers Chemical Methods in Penetration Enhancement.* Springer, Berlin, Heidelberg.

Rancan, F., Papakostas, D., Hadam, S., Hackbarth, S., Delair, T., Primard, C., Verrier, B., Sterry, W., Blume-Peytavi, U., Vogt, A., 2009 Aug. Investigation of polylactic acid (PLA) nanoparticles as drug delivery systems for local dermatotherapy. *Pharm Res.* 26(8), 2027–2036.

Redelmeier, T., Kitson, N., 1999. Dermatological Applications of Liposomes. In: Janoff, A.S. (ed) *Liposomes. Rational Design.* Marcell Dekker, pp. 283–307.

Rizwan, M., Aqil, M., Talegaonkar, S., Azeem, A., Sultana, Y., Ali, A., 2009 Jun. Enhanced transdermal drug delivery techniques: an extensive review of patents. *Recent Pat. Drug Deliv. Formul.* 3(2), 105–124.

Roberts, M.S., Pugh, W.J., Hadgraft, J., 1996. Epidermal permeability-penetrant structure relationships. 2. The effect of H-bonding groups in penetrants on their diffusion through the stratum corneum. *Int. J. Pharm.* 132, 23–32.

Rouse, J.G., Yang, J., Ryman-Rasmussen, J.P., Barron, A.R., Monteiro-Riviere, N.A., 2007 Jan. Effects of mechanical flexion on the penetration of fullerene amino acid-derivatized peptide nanoparticles through skin. *Nano Lett.* 7(1), 155–160.

Schaefer, H., Redelmeier, T.E., 1996. *Skin Barrier: Principles of Percutaneous Absorption.* Karger, Basel, New York.

Schaefer, H., Lademann, J., 2001. The role of follicular penetration. A differential view. *Skin Pharmacol. Appl. Skin Physiol.* 14 Suppl 1, 23–27.

Schätzlein, A., Cevc, G., 1998 Apr. Non-uniform cellular packing of the stratum corneum and permeability barrier function of intact skin: a high-resolution confocal laser scanning microscopy study using highly deformable vesicles (Transfersomes). *Br. J. Dermatol.* 138(4), 583–592.

Scheuplein, R.J., 1967 Jan. Mechanism of percutaneous absorption. II. Transient diffusion and the relative importance of various routes of skin penetration. *J. Invest. Dermatol.* 48(1), 79–88.

Schmidt, R.R., 1992. Ceramides for Liposomes. In: Braun-Falco, O., Korting, H.C., Maibach, H.I. (eds) *Liposome Dermatics.* Springer-Verlag, Berlin, 44–56.

Shah, D.K., Khandavilli, S., Panchagnula, R., 2008. Alteration of skin hydration and its barrier function by vehicle and permeation enhancers: a study using TGA, FTIR, TEWL and drug permeation as markers. *Methods Find. Exp. Clin. Pharmacol.* 30, 499–512.

Shim, J., Seok, K.H., Park, W.S., Han, S.H., Kim, J., Chang, I.S., 2004. Transdermal delivery of minoxidil with block copolymer nanoparticles. *J. Control. Release* 97, 477–484.

Sugiyama-Nakagiri, Y., Akiyama, M., Shimizu, H., 2006. Hair follicle stem cell targeted gene transfer and reconstitution system. *Gene Ther.* 13, 732–737.

Toll, R., Jacobi, U., Richter, H., Lademann, J., Schaefer, H., Blume-Peytavi, U., 2004. Penetration profile of microspheres in follicular targeting of terminal hair follicles. *J. Invest. Dermatol.* 123, 168–176.

Uche, L.E., Gooris, G.S., Beddoes, C.M., Bouwstra, J.A., 2019 Jul 1. New insight into phase behavior and permeability of skin lipid models based on sphingosine and phytosphingosine ceramides. *Biochim. Biophys. Acta Biomembr.* 1861(7), 1317–1328.

Van Kuijk-Meuwissen, M.E., Mougin, L., Junginger, H.E., Bouwstra, J.A., 1998 Dec 4. Application of vesicles to rat skin *in vivo*: a confocal laser scanning microscopy study. *J Control Release.* 56(1-3), 189–196.

Vogt, A., Blume-Peytavi, U., 2003. Biology of the human hair follicle. *New Knowl. Clin. Significance. Hautarzt* 54, 692–698.

Vogt, A., Mandt, N., Lademann, J., Schaefer, H., Blume-Peytavi, U., 2005. Follicular targeting – a promising tool in selective dermatotherapy. *J. Invest. Dermatol. Symp. Proc.* 10, 252–255.

Vogt, A., Combadiere, B., Hadam, S., Stieler, K.M., Lademann, J., Schaefer, H., Autran, B., Sterry, W., Blume-Peytavi, U., 2006. 40 nm, but not 750 or 1,500 nm, nanoparticles enter epidermal CD1a+ cells after transcutaneous application on human skin. *J. Invest. Dermatol.* 126, 1316–1322.

Vogt, A., Mahe, B., Costagliola, D., Bonduelle, O., Hadam, S., Schaefer, G., Schaefer, H., Katlama, C., Sterry, W., Autran, B., Blume-Peytavi, U., Combadiere, B.,

2008. Transcutaneous anti-influenza vaccination promotes both CD4 and CD8 T cell immune responses in humans. *J. Immunol.* 180, 1482–1489.

Wang, F., Chen, Y., Benson, H.A.E., 2008. Formulation of nano and micro PLGA particles of the model peptide insulin: preparation, characterization, stability and deposition in human skin. *Open Drug Delivery J.* 2, 1–9.

Wertz, P.W., 1992. Liposome Dermatics: Chemical Aspects of the Skin Lipid Approach. In: Braun-Falco, O., Korting, H.C., Maibach, H.I. (eds) *Liposome Dermatics*. Springer-Verlag, Berlin, pp. 38–43.

Wertz P.W., 2015. Epidermal Lipids and the Intercellular Pathway. In: Dragicevic, N., Maibach, H. (eds) *Percutaneous Penetration Enhancers Chemical Methods in Penetration Enhancement*. Springer, Berlin, Heidelberg.

Wertz, P.W., Swartzendruber, D.C., Madison, K.C., Downing, D.T., 1987. Composition and morphology of epidermal cyst lipids. *J. Invest Dermatol.* 89, 419–425.

Wertz, P., Norlén, L., 2003. "Confidence Intervals" for the "true" lipid compositions of the human skin barrier? In: Forslind, B., Lindberg, M. (eds) *Skin, Hair, and Nails. Structure and Function.* Marcel Dekker Inc., 85-106. Biochim. Biophys. Acta 304:265–275.

Williams, A.C., 2003. *Transdermal and Topical Drug Delivery From Theory To Clinical Practice.* Pharmaceutical Press, London; Chicago.

Wilkes, G.L., Brown, I.A., Wildnauer, R.H., 1973 Aug. The biomechanical properties of skin. *CRC Crit. Rev. Bioeng.* 1(4), 453–495.

Williams, A.C., Barry, B.W., 1991 Jan. Terpenes and the lipid-protein-partitioning theory of skin penetration enhancement. *Pharm. Res.* 8(1), 17–24.

Williams, A.C., Barry, B.W., 2004 Mar 27. Penetration enhancers. *Adv. Drug Deliv. Rev.* 56(5), 603–618.

Williams, M.L., 1984. The dynamics of desquamation. Lessons to be learned from the ichthyoses. *Am J Dermatopathol.* 6(4), 381–385. doi: 10.1097/00000372-1984 08000-00013. PMID: 6388396.

Zheng, Z., Diaz-Arévalo, D., Guan, H., Zeng, M., 2018. Noninvasive vaccination against infectious diseases. *Hum Vaccin Immunother.* 14(7), 1717–1733. doi: 10.1080/21645515.2018.1461296. Epub 2018 May 17. PMID: 29624470; PMCID: PMC6067898.

Zbytovska, J., Vavrova, K., Kiselev, M.A., Lessieur, P., Wartewig, S., Neubert, R.H.H., 2009. The effects of transdermal permeation enhancers on thermotropic phase behaviour of a stratum corneum lipid model. *Colloid Surface A* 351, 30–37.

Lipid-Based Vesicles (Liposomes) as Skin Delivery Systems

2

2.1 COMPOSITION AND CLASSIFICATION OF LIPOSOMES

Liposomes (lipid-based vesicles) represent the first and most studied vesicular carriers for the delivery of drugs into the skin. The liposome story began with a paper in 1964, published in the *Journal of Molecular Biology*, in which Bangham and Horne showed electron microscopic images of multilamellar phospholipid vesicles (Bangham and Horne, 1964). The term liposomes, derived from two Greek words "lipos" (fat) and "soma" (body) was proposed for the description of lipid vesicles in 1968 (Sessa and Weissmann, 1968).

Liposomes represent colloidal particles, typically consisting of phospholipids and cholesterol, both being the major structural components of conventional liposomes, and aqueous medium (water or buffer solution). The amphipathic nature of phospholipids and their analogs render them the ability to form closed concentric bilayers in the presence of water. When phospholipids are exposed to an aqueous environment, interactions between themselves (hydrophilic interactions between polar headgroups and Van der Waals' interactions between hydrocarbon chains) and with water (hydrophilic interactions, hydrophobic effect) lead to the spontaneous formation of closed bilayers (Bangham et al., 1965; Lautenschläger, 2006; Siler-Marinkovic, 2016). As to

DOI: 10.1201/9781003187332-2

liposomes' drug carrier ability, they can encapsulate hydrophilic drugs within the aqueous regions, and incorporate lipophilic drugs within the lipid bilayers (Figure 2.1).

Liposomes are typically composed of natural phospholipids (PL) due to their low cost and toxicological considerations, and the most used are phosphatidylcholine (PC), phosphatidylethanolamine (PE), phosphatidylserine (PS), phosphatidyl inositol (PI) and phosphatidyl glycerol (PG) (Figure 2.2). However, the following synthetic phospholipids have also been used: dioleoylphosphatidylcholine (DOPC), distearoylphosphatidylcholine (DSPC), dipalmitoylphosphatidylcholine (DPPC), dioleoylphosphatidylethanolamine (DOPE) and distearoylphosphatidylethanolamine (DSPE), but less often compared to natural phospholipids (especially egg PC (EPC) and soya PC (SPC)). Cholesterol (CHOL) is added to improve the stability of the bilayers as it reduces the bilayers' permeability and drug leakage (Bennett et al., 2009). However, CHOL increases the rigidity of liposomes, as it increases the phospholipid bilayers' phase transition temperature (T_m), from the gel state to the liquid crystalline state, which further has a negative impact on the penetration enhancing ability of liposomes (Jain et al., 2015). Liposomes may contain also other ingredients, such as surfactants/ethanol/terpenes to increase their deformability (Cevc et al., 2008a; Touitou et al., 2000; Dragicevic-Curic et al., 2008), stearylamine and diacetyl phosphate to impart either a negative or a positive surface charge to liposomes (Dragicevic-Curic et al., 2010), etc. Further, in order to decrease the oxidation of phospholipids, besides neutral pH buffers also antioxidants can be incorporated into liposomes.

The lipid composition, type of lipid, drug-lipid ratio, concentration and type of surface charge imparting compound, etc. have an impact on the physicochemical properties and skin penetration enhancing ability of liposomes (Bhatia et al., 2004; Puglia et al., 2010).

Physico-chemical properties are used to characterize liposomes. Size distribution, homogeneity, lamellarity, phase transition temperature (T_m), drug encapsulation efficiency (EE%), and zeta potential are monitored during their physical stability assessment, while drug content, pH value, oxidation index, hydrolysis rate, are determined in terms of investigating their chemical stability. Monitoring these liposomes' parameters during their stability investigation is of crucial importance, as the shelf life of liposomes is determined by their physical and chemical stability. Besides physical instability (expressed as a fusion of vesicles, aggregation, and encapsulation capacity reduction) and chemical instability (expressed as oxidation of unsaturated fatty acids in the lipid bilayer, lipid hydrolysis, and degradation of the drug, which may lead to the disruption of liposomes' membranes and leaking of encapsulated materials), also microbiological instability may occur as liposomes are an excellent medium for bacterial growth (Šiler-Marinkovic, 2016).

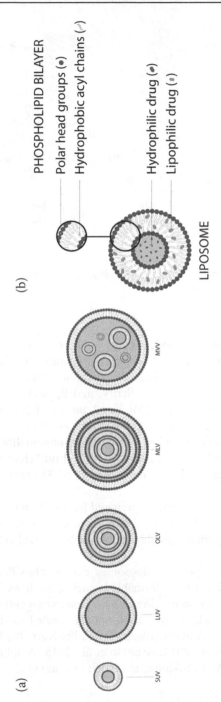

FIGURE 2.1   Schematic illustration of a) the liposome structure and b) liposome classification.

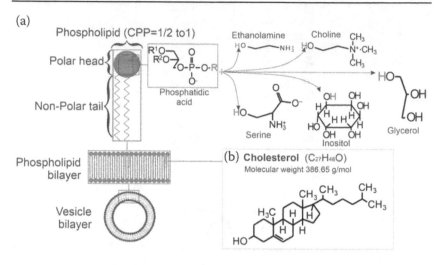

FIGURE 2.2 Phospholipids and cholesterol as constituents of liposomes (Castañeda-Reyes et al., 2020).

Liposomes can be classified in many ways, e.g. dependent on their lamellarity (number of phospholipid bilayers), preparation method, composition (tailored according to their application indication), etc. The most common classification is based on their lamellarity, and liposomes can be classified into: multilamellar large vesicles (MLV, >1 µm or >0.5 µm), oligolamellar vesicles (OLV, 0.1–1 µm), small unilamellar vesicles (SUV, 20–100 nm), medium-sized unilamellar vesicles (MUV), large unilamellar vesicles (LUV, >100 nm) and giant unilamellar vesicles (GUV, >1 µm) (Kriftner, 1992). Also multivesicular vesicles can be obtained (MVV, >1000 nm) (Lautenschläger, 2006) (Figure 2.1).

Liposomes are most commonly prepared by the "film method" and MLV are obtained (Rosoft, 1988; New, 1990; Lautenschläger, 2006). For more details regarding preparation methods, the reader should refer to Patil and Jadhav (2014).

Based on their composition liposomes can be classified into: conventional liposomes and elastic/deformable vesicles, such as Transfersomes® (Idea AG, Germany), ethosomes, invasomes, penetration enhancer-containing vesicles (PEVs), etc., which have been widely studied as drug carriers for dermal and transdermal delivery (Elsabahy and Foldvari, 2013a; Priyanka and Singh, 2014; Zhang et al., 2014; Ascenso et al., 2015; Avadhani et al., 2017; Caddeo et al., 2018; Abd El-Alim et al., 2019; Hussain et al., 2020), as well as long-circulating PEG-coated liposomes (sterically stabilized (Stealth®) liposomes) used for parenteral drug delivery.

Liposomes have been widely used for dermal drug delivery due to their numerous advantages over conventional formulations, since they may: (1) be carriers for both hydrophilic and lipophilic drugs, (2) solubilize drugs with low water solubility, (3) improve the skin accumulation of the drug, while reducing systemic drug absorption and associated adverse effects, (4) form drug depots in the skin with controlled sustained drug release, (5) provide targeted drug delivery to skin appendages, (6) increase the chemical stability of drugs (especially photostability) (El Maghraby et al., 2008; El Maghraby and Williams, 2009; Sinico and Fadda, 2009). In addition, liposomes are biodegradable, non-toxic, with low allergic potential, and are generally recognized as safe (GRAS status) by the Food and Drug Administration (FDA) (Parnham, 1992; Raza et al., 2013; Rukavina et al., 2018).

However, liposomes have not entered the market of topical preparations in a large number. The main problems limiting the manufacture and development of liposomal preparations have been: stability issues, reproducibility, scalability of the manufacturing process, sterilization method, residual organic solvent in the drug product, low drug entrapment, and high production costs (Thoma and Jocham, 1992; Sharma and Sharma, 1997). Although there are only a few commercial topical liposomal products, there is a considerable body of research on this topic (El Maghraby et al., 2008; de Leeuw et al., 2009; El Maghraby and Williams, 2009; Sinico and Fadda, 2009; Jain et al., 2015; Sala et al., 2018).

Regarding transdermal drug delivery, it is rarely achieved by conventional liposomes as they are mainly confined to the *stratum corneum* (SC) (El Maghraby et al., 2008).

2.1.1 Physicochemical Properties of Liposomes Influencing Their Penetration-Enhancing Ability

a. **Influence of lipid composition**
   The key parameter of liposomes affecting drug permeation across the SC and the interactions with the SC is the thermodynamic state of the bilayers, which is expressed by the T_m of liposomes' bilayers. Bilayers of vesicles are depending on their lipid composition either in a liquid crystalline state, which is characterized by the fluid state of bilayers or in a gel state, which is characterized by rigid bilayers (Riaz et al., 1989; Dragicevic-Curic et al., 2011).

Increased drug penetration from conventional liquid-state vesicles compared to gel state vesicles has been reported for a lot of compounds, such as progesterone (Knepp et al., 1988, 1990), CsA (Dowton et al.,1993), triamcinolone acetonide (TRMA) (Yu and Liao, 1996), fluorescein (Perez-Cullell et al., 2000), enoxacin (Fang et al., 2001a), etc. Van Kuijk-Meuwissen et al. (1998a,b) confirmed *in vitro* in human skin and *in vivo* in rats the importance of the thermodynamic state of vesicles, showing that the lipophilic fluorescent label incorporated in gel-state conventional liposomes or micelles did not penetrate into the skin as deeply as the label applied in liquid-state conventional liposomes. In addition, among liquid-state vesicles, the vesicles with flexible bilayers (containing a single-chain surfactant in bilayers) showed the highest penetration into the dermis. These results were confirmed by El Maghraby et al. (1999, 2001a), which led to the development of a wide range of different deformable/flexible vesicles containing in their phospholipid bilayers edge activators imparting deformability to the bilayers.

It has also been shown that the mode of liposomes application is of great importance. Non-occlusive application of liposomes results in higher drug penetration compared to the occlusive application (Cevc and Blume, 1992; Cevc, 1996; El Maghraby and Williams, 2009; Van Kuijk-Meuwissen et al., 1998a).

b. **Influence of particle size**

It was assumed that if intact liposomes penetrated the skin, their size would influence drug delivery through the skin. Hence, smaller vesicles would lead to a higher drug disposition in the lower skin layers than when the drug was applied in larger vesicles. Results of different studies investigating the influence of particle size on the penetration-enhancing ability of liposomes are represented in Table 2.1. Some of the findings were in favor of the absence of intact vesicle penetration across the skin as there was no increase of drug penetration upon decreasing liposomes' size (Egbaria et al., 1990b; Hofland et al., 1994; El Maghraby et al., 1999). However, there were also studies reporting that there might be a favorable particle size for optimal drug delivery (Yu and Liao, 1996; Esposito et al., 1998; Gabrijelcic et al., 1994; Verma et al., 2003a).

c. **Surface charge**

Many researchers have outlined that drug penetration can be influenced by modifying the surface charge of liposomes (Table 2.1). Most of the authors demonstrated a higher drug penetration into/through the skin from positively charged

TABLE 2.1 Influence of physico-chemical properties of liposomes on their penetration-enhancing ability

PARAMETER INVESTIGATED	FORMULATION	DRUG	INDICATION	CONDITION	OUTCOME	REFERENCE
Particle size	MLV LUV (SCL and PL)	Cylosporine A (CsA)	Alopecia areata	in vitro	MLV, being of higher particle size delivered a higher total amount of CsA in the deeper SC and deeper skin layers than LUV, being of smaller particle size.	Egbaria et al. (1990b)
	PC/CHOL/cholesteryl sulfate liposomes 60– 600 nm	CsA	Alopecia areata	in vitro hairless mouse, hamster and pig skin	Intermediate particle size of 300 nm, provided both the highest reservoirs in the deeper skin layers, as well as the highest drug concentration in the receiver.	Du Plessis 1994
	Liposomes of different particle size	Estradiol	Hormone replacement therapy	in vitro human skin	No penetration enhancement with SUV.	Hofland et al. (1994)

(Continued)

TABLE 2.1 (Continued) Influence of physico-chemical properties of liposomes on their penetration-enhancing ability

PARAMETER INVESTIGATED	FORMULATION	DRUG	INDICATION	CONDITION	OUTCOME	REFERENCE
	Liposomes of different particle size	Estradiol	Hormone replacement therapy	in vitro human skin	SUV (124–138 nm) were as effective as LMLV (557 nm)	El Maghraby et al. (1999)
	SUV and MLV with negative surface charge	TRMA	Corticosteroid therapy against skin inflammation	in vitro rat skin	SUV provided a significantly higher permeation of TRMA than the MLV of same charge	Yu and Liao (1996)
	Liposomes of different particle size	Methyl nicotinate		in vitro human skin	Permeability coefficient of methyl nicotinate was inversely related to the liposome size	Esposito et al. (1998)
	Liposomes of different particle size	Hydrophilic compound		pig ear skin in vitro	penetration of a hydrophilic compound was 100-fold higher when applied in	Gabrijelcic et al. (1994)

	Liposomes of different particle size	Lipophilic and a hydrophilic fluorescent label		In vitro Human skin	small REV than in large MLV Smallest liposomes provided the highest label penetration into the skin	Verma et al. (2003a)
Surface charge	Liposomes of positive, negative and neutral surface charge	Retinoic acid	Retinoid	*in vitro* human skin	Higher skin permeation of retinoic acid from positively charged liposomes compared to negatively charged liposomes, showing similar permeation as neutral liposomes	Montenegro et al. (1996)
	Liposomes of positive, negative and neutral surface charge	rhodamine B	model drug	*in vitro* in rat skin	Higher skin permeability of rhodamine B from positively charged	Katahira et al. (1999)

(Continued)

TABLE 2.1 (Continued) Influence of physico-chemical properties of liposomes on their penetration-enhancing ability

PARAMETER INVESTIGATED	FORMULATION	DRUG	INDICATION	CONDITION	OUTCOME	REFERENCE
	Liposomes of different surface charge	Methyl nicotinate (MN)		in vivo	liposomes compared to negatively charged liposomes Higher release of MN from neutral and negatively charged liposomes compared to positively charged.	Puglia et al. (2005)
	Liposomes of different surface charge	Amphotericin B		in vitro in rat skin	Positively charged liposomes provided the highest drug flux through the SC, and negatively charged liposomes through the viable epidermis.	Manosroi et al. (2004)

Liposomes of different surface charge	Acyclovir palmitate	In vitro	skin retention of acyclovir palmitate from positively charged liposomes was higher than from other	Liu et al. (2004)
Flexible vesicles of different surface charge	Low molecular weight heparin	in vitro in vivo	Cationic flexible vesicles induced a significantly greater permeation and penetration into the deeper skin layers compared to neutral and anionic vesicles.	Song and Kim (2006)
Liposomes and niosomes of different surface charge	Enoxacin	In vitro	Negatively charged liposomes and niosomes reduced the permeation of enoxacin through the skin.	Fang et al. (2001a)

(Continued)

TABLE 2.1 (Continued)   Influence of physico-chemical properties of liposomes on their penetration-enhancing ability

PARAMETER INVESTIGATED	FORMULATION	DRUG	INDICATION	CONDITION	OUTCOME	REFERENCE
	Liposomes of different surface charge	Clindamycine phosphate		in vitro mice skin	Cationic liposomes provided higher clindamycine phosphate permeation through the skin than neutral and negatively charged liposomes.	Shanmugam et al. (2009)
	Liposomes coated with two cationic polymers, chitosan and Eudragit® EPO (poly(butyl methacrylate-co- (2-dimethylaminoethyl) methacrylate-co-methyl methacrylate))	Minoxidil and acyclovir		In vitro	Coated cationic liposomes led to a higher skin diffusion of both drugs compared to uncoated liposomes.	Hasanovic et al. (2010)
	Surface-charged flexible liposomes	Temoporfin (mTHPC)	Photodynamic therapy (PDT)	In vitro Human skin	Cationic flexible liposomes delivered the highest mTHPC-amount into the SC and deeper skin layers.	Dragicevic-Curic et al. (2010)

liposomes compared to neutral and negatively charged liposomes (Montenegro et al., 1996; Katahira et al. 1999; Fang et al., 2001a; Manosroi et al., 2004; Liu et al., 2004; Shanmugam et al., 2009; Hasanovic et al., 2010). They proposed that the electrostatic interaction between the negatively charged skin surface (Burnette and Ongpipattanakul, 1987) and the positively charged liposomes could promote drug penetration and its consequent rapid depletion by the bloodstream in the vascularized section of the skin. Higher skin penetration of drugs encapsulated into cationic vesicles was also seen for flexible cationic vesicles (Song and Kim, 2006; Dragicevic-Curic et al., 2010). However, some authors found the opposite, i.e. they demonstrated *in vitro* and *in vivo* the capability of negatively charged liposomes to increase the permeation rate of different model drugs into/through the skin (Ogiso 2001, El-Alim 2019; Puglia et al., 2005).

2.2 LIPOSOMES AS SKIN DRUG DELIVERY SYSTEMS

2.2.1 Liposomes as Topical Drug Delivery Systems (Localizing Effects)

For dermato-pharmacotherapy, there is a need for a drug delivery system that enhances the penetration of the active ingredient into the skin, localizes the drug at the site of action at therapeutic levels, and reduces percutaneous absorption. Conventional liposomes have been used since the 1980s as drug carrier systems for topical delivery, as they have the potential to *enhance drug penetration into the skin* (El Maghraby et al., 2000a; Belhaj et al., 2017; Joseph et al., 2018; Mostafa et al., 2018), *improve therapeutic effectiveness* (Mura et al., 2007; Oh et al., 2011; Manca et al., 2016; Jeong et al., 2017), *decrease side-effects* (Seth et al., 2004) and act as a *local depot*s (Schreier and Bouwstra, 1994). Conventional liposomes are the most commonly and extensively studied vesicle carriers for dermal drug delivery.

The potential value of liposomes was first recognized by Mezei and Gulasekharam (1980). They reported that DPPC:CHOL vesicles increased the amount of the *corticosteroid* drug TRMA in the epidermis and dermis *in vivo* in rabbits by 4 to 5-fold and reduced percutaneous absorption compared to a conventional ointment. Similar findings were observed in numerous studies, conducted from the 1980s to about 2000. Liposomes have been shown to significantly enhance skin delivery of drugs, thus forming local depots with sustained release of a variety of drugs, such as hydrocortisone (Kim et al., 1997), TRMA (Monti et al., 2004), interferon (Egbaria et al., 1990a), cyclosporine A (Egbaria et al., 1990b), dyphylline (Touitou et al., 1992), caffeine (Touitou et al., 1994a), tetracaine (Gesztes and Mezei, 1988), lidocaine (Foldvari et al., 1990), tretinoin (Touitou et al., 1994b; Manosroi et al., 2004), dithranol (Agarwal et al., 2001), 5-fluorouracil (El Maghraby et al., 2001a), tacrolimus (Erdogan et al., 2002), etc. Generally, in the case of high penetrating drugs, such as progesterone, trihexyphenidyl hydrochloride, and caffeine, conventional liposomes induce lower drug permeation than the control, however, higher drug retention in the skin, which is desired (Knepp et al., 1988; Touitou et al., 1994a; Dayan and Touitou, 2000). Liposomes greatly enhanced the penetration of even minimally permeable drugs into human skin *in vitro*, such as the unfractionated macromolecule heparin (Betz et al., 2001). As promising results were obtained, conventional liposomes continued to be intensively studied, and studies after the year 2000 introduced new drug candidates for liposomal encapsulation for the treatment of various skin disorders/infections, *alopecia areata*, *acne vulgaris*, psoriasis, inflammatory diseases, anti-aging treatments, skin cancers, cutaneous leishmaniasis, etc. (Table 2.2). Liposomes encapsulating various active compounds have been used with high therapeutic effectiveness in wound healing and skin regeneration (Wang et al., 2019) as they effectively cover wounds and create a moist environment on wound surface after application, which is very conducive to wound healing (Manca et al., 2016). The numerous studies which are described in Table 2.2. reflect the *localizing effect* of liposomes, resulting in the formation of large drug reservoirs in the skin, which can be used for the local treatment of skin disorders.

2.2.2 Liposomes as Drug Delivery Systems Targeting the Skin Appendages

The pilosebaceous route also contributes significantly to topical and transdermal delivery (Lauer, 1999; Patzelt and Lademann, 2015). The potential of liposomes to target the skin appendages, especially the pilosebaceous unit (hair follicle, hair shaft, and sebaceous gland) has been studied in detail (Lauer, 1999; El Maghraby et al., 2004; Patzelt and Lademann, 2015) as it could be beneficial for treating hair follicle-associated disorders, like acne vulgaris, alopecia areata, and some cancers, as well as for vaccination, gene

TABLE 2.2 Conventional liposomes as carriers for dermal drug delivery

FORMULATION	DRUG	INDICATION	CONDITIONS	OUTCOME	REFERENCE
Liposomes	Tamoxifen,	Breast cancer, skin disorders		Liposomes provided significantly higher skin permeation of tamoxifen (drug flux 63.67 µg/cm²/h and 59.87 µg/cm²/h for liposomal suspension and liposomal gel) as compared to the solution (21.65 µg/cm²/h) and carbomer gel (24.55 µg/cm²/h) containing tamoxifen. Higher drug skin retention was achieved with liposomal formulations compared to non-liposomal formulations.	Bhatia et al. (2004)

(Continued)

TABLE 2.2 (Continued) Conventional liposomes as carriers for dermal drug delivery

FORMULATION	DRUG	INDICATION	CONDITIONS	OUTCOME	REFERENCE
Liposomes	Polyvinyl-pyrrolidone (PVP)-iodine	antiseptic and anti-inflammatory agent	Patients with acne vulgaris, atopic dermatitis, impetigo contagiosa and rosacea received 3% PVP-iodine hydrogel for ≤4 weeks	PVP-iodine hydrogel has shown to be an effective treatment for inflammatory skin conditions associated with bacterial colonization.	Augustin et al. (2017)
Different liposomes	Azithromycin	Methicillin-resistant *Staphylococcus aureus* (MRSA) strains infections	In vitro	Liposomes delivered azithromycin into the skin more efficiently than the control	Rukavina et al. (2018)
Liposomes	Berberine and curcumin	Antibacterial agents for methicillin-resistant *Staphylococcus aureus* (MRSA) infections	In vitro	Co-encapsulation of berberine and curcumin in liposomes decreased their MIC by 87% and 96%, respectively, as compared to their free forms; inhibited growth of MRSA and	Bhatia et al. (2021)

Multilayered liposomes properly coated with polyelectrolytes of anionic sodium hyaluronate (HA) and cationic chitosan (CH)	*quercetin*	*antioxidant*	*in vitro*	prevented biofilm formation to a higher extent compared to free drugs; reduced intracellular infection to 77% and the production of pro-inflammatory cytokines by macrophages. Therapeutic effectiveness of novel liposomes was 5-fold higher than that of clindamycin. Negatively charged (HA-CH)-liposomes and positively charged CH-liposomes revealed similar skin permeability, which was superior	Jeon et al. (2015)

(Continued)

TABLE 2.2 (Continued) Conventional liposomes as carriers for dermal drug delivery

FORMULATION	DRUG	INDICATION	CONDITIONS	OUTCOME	REFERENCE
				to that of uncoated liposomes.	
Liposomes	Co-incorporated quercetin and resveratrol	Antioxidants	In vivo	Remarkable amelioration of the tissue damage in skin lesions, with a significant reduction of edema and leukocyte infiltration	Caddeo et al. (2018)
Novel liposomes with hydrogel core of silk fibroin	fibroblast growth factor (bFGF)	Wound healing	In vitro In vivo	The liposomal encapsulation improved the stability of bFGF in wound fuids and maintained cell proliferation activity with respect to free bFGF and traditional liposomes, and accelerated wound healing	Xu et al. (2017)

Liposomes	Madecassoside	Wound healing	In vitro In vivo	Liposomes enhanced permeation and distribution of the active substance in into the skin and exhibited superior burn wound healing effect.	Li et al. (2016)
Liposomes, niosomes and propylene glycol-water-ethanol solution	*Minoxidil*	*Alopecia*	*in vitro* human skin	The greatest skin accumulation was obtained with non-dialyzed vesicular formulations.	Mura et al. (2007)
	Adapalene	*Acne vulgaris*	In vitro	liposomal encapsulation revealed enhanced drug delivery into the skin and hair follicles	Kumar and Banga (2016), Ingebrigtsen et al. (2017)
Liposomes (phosphatidylcholine, cholesterol), ethosomes (phosphatidylcholine, ethanol), solid lipid nanoparticles	Tretinoin	Acne vulgaris, psoriasis, skin cancers, etc	Ex vivo permeation in mouse skin, anti-psoriatic activity in mouse tail model	The highest permeation flux was provided by NLC, while the highest drug retention was	Raza et al. (2013)

(Continued)

TABLE 2.2 (Continued) Conventional liposomes as carriers for dermal drug delivery

FORMULATION	DRUG	INDICATION	CONDITIONS	OUTCOME	REFERENCE
(phosphatidylcholine, polysorbate (Tween® 80), glyceryl dibehenate (Compritol® 888), ethanol) and nanostructured lipid carriers (NLC) (phosphatidylcholine, Tween® 80, Compritol® 888, ethanol, isopropyl myristate), incorporated into a gel				obtained by the liposomal gel. Liposomal gel was found to be efficient for the treatment of superficial skin disorders, such as psoriasis.	
Lipase- sensitive liposomes by coating of lipase-sensitive moieties onto conventional liposomes	Erythromycin	Antibiotic		Lipase-sensitive liposomes enhanced antimicrobial effect in treating *Acne vulgaris.*	Jeong et al. (2017)
Liposomal gel	*Methotrexate combined with menthol in gel*	*Psoriasis*	*ex vivo* rat skin in vivo anti-psoriatic effectiveness in rat tail model	Liposomal gel enhanced drug penetration into rat skin and caused drug retention in the skin and skin appendages. Anti-	Nagle et al. (2011)

Cationic and anionic liposomes formulated into a liposomal gel	*Psoralen*	*Psoriasis*	*In vitro* *In vivo* imiquimod induced psoriatic plaque model	psoriatic effectiveness was confirmed. Liposomal formulation provided higher psoralen penetration into the skin and a 5-fold increase in permeation of psoralen compared to drug solution. Liposomal gels reduced the symptoms of psoriasis and levels of key psoriatic cytokines.	Doppalapudi et al. (2017)
Cationic liposomes formulated into a liposomal gel.	Cyclosporine (CsA)	Psoriasis	*In vivo* imiquimod induced psoriatic plaque model	Liposomal gels reduced the symptoms of psoriasis and levels of key psoriatic cytokines.	Walunj et al. (2020)
Liposomes and ethosomes formulated into a gel	*Anthralin*	Psoriasis	Clinical efficacy and safety in	After treatment, mean PASI change	Fathalla et al. (2020)

(Continued)

TABLE 2.2 (Continued) Conventional liposomes as carriers for dermal drug delivery

FORMULATION	DRUG	INDICATION	CONDITIONS	OUTCOME	REFERENCE
			patients having psoriasis	was -68.66% and -81.84% for liposomes and ethosomes.	
Liposomal gel	Diclofenac	Non-steroidal anti-inflammatory drug (NSAID)	Double blind randomized, placebo controlled, clinical trial in patients with knee osteoarthritis.	Diclofenac-loaded liposomal gel, was superior in relieving/improving the symptoms of knee osteoarthritis (pain, stiffness, physical function), in comparison to placebo and marketed Diclofenac gel (Voveran® Emulgel®, Novartis).	Bhatia et al. (2020)
Stratum corneum lipid liposomes (SCLLs)	Naproxen	Non-steroidal anti-inflammatory drug (NSAID)	In vitro	SCLLs enhanced skin delivery of naproxen, whilst PC/CHOL liposomes promoted	Puglia et al. (2010)

System	Drug/agent	Activity	Study type	Results	Reference
Liposomes incorporated into a chitosan gel	Thymoquinone (major constituent of *Nigella sativa* oil)	Anti-inflammatory agent	*in vivo* carrageenan-induced paw edema in rats	naproxen permeation through the skin. Liposomal gel showed *in vivo* in rats, superior anti-inflammatory activity over the thymoquinone-chitosan gel, and a comparable effect to the marketed indomethacin gel.	Mostafa et al. (2018)
Liposomes	*Curcumin*	Anti-inflammatory, antioxidant and antibacterial agent	*ex vivo*	Liposomes provided an improved curcumin deposition in the epidermis, which acts as a drug reservoir.	Campani et al. (2020)
Liposomes	*Ascorbic acid*	*Antioxidant agent; increases collagen synthesis*	*In vitro*	Negatively charged liposomes, favored skin retention, showing a 2.6- and 5.1-fold higher accumulation in epidermis and	Maione-Silva et al. (2019)

(Continued)

TABLE 2.2 (Continued) Conventional liposomes as carriers for dermal drug delivery

FORMULATION	DRUG	INDICATION	CONDITIONS	OUTCOME	REFERENCE
				dermis, respectively, compared to the aqueous solution of ascorbic acid. They improved keratinocytes regeneration.	
Non-coated and polysaccharide-coated liposomes (Ionosomes™)	caffeine, hexapeptide	Anti-ageing	In vitro	Both types of liposomes improved the penetration of both actives into the skin.	Belhaj et al. (2017)
Liposomes formulated into a gel	Temoporfin (mTHPC)	PDT of psoriasis, skin cancer, etc.	In vitro Human skin	Liposomal gel delivered sufficiently high amounts of mTHPC to the SC and deeper skin layers.	Dragicevic-Curic et al. (2009, 2010)
DPPC liposomes	5-ALA	PDT of epithelial skin cancers	Ex vivo, mice in vivo	Liposomes provided higher penetration of 5-ALA compared to free	Lin et al. (2016)

| Liposomes with different drug concentration | Amphotericin B | Cutaneous leishmaniasis | *in vitro* on L. major and L. tropica, *in vivo* on L. major infection in BALB/c mice | 5-ALA. Liposoms enhanced protoporphyrin IX (PpIX) accumulation only in tumor tissue, in melanoma xenograft models. After 8 and 12 weeks of treatment with Amphotericin B (0.4%)-loaded liposomes, the parasite was completely cleared from the skin site of infection and spleens, respectively. | Jaafari et al. (2019) |

therapy, and for accelerated systemic delivery via transport through the shunt pathway (Lauer, 1999; Verma et al., 2004; Castro and Ferreira, 2008).

It has been shown in numerous studies that liposomes provided better drug targeting to the pilosebaceous unit (higher drug deposition in the hair follicle) than aqueous, aqueous/ethanolic and other solutions, e.g. for the fluorescent dye calcein and the pigment melanin (Li et al., 1992, 1993a, Li and Hoffman, 1997), fluorescent dye carboxyfluorescein (CF) (Lieb et al., 1992), γ-interferon (Du Plessis et al., 1992), clindamycin (Škalko et al., 1992), cimetidine (Lieb et al., 1994), finasteride (Tabbakhian et al., 2006). Li et al. (1993b) showed high deposition of deoxyribonucleic acid (DNA) into the hair follicle of mice *in vitro* upon entrapment into liposomes, which could be used for gene therapy (Hoffman, 2005).

Jung et al. (2006) showed by confocal laser scanning microscopy (CLSM) that liposomes provided a higher penetration depth of the hydrophilic CF and lipophilic curcumin than free dye solutions. The relative penetration depth of the dyes, applied as solutions averaged 30% of the full follicle length, whereas amphoteric and cationic liposomes reached an average relative penetration depth of 70% of the full hair follicle length, as cationic vesicles would bind in an ion-exchange manner to the negatively charged surface of the SC and the hair, and consequently reach greater accumulation. Keeping in mind the high penetration depth of liposomes in pig ear skin and the absolute length of the human hair follicle, all applied liposomal formulations would be able in human skin to act as a follicular drug delivery system (Jung et al., 2006). The infundibula of porcine hair follicles on average extend to approximately 50% of the follicle length, as seen in this study (Jung et al., 2006), while the infundibula of human hair follicles extend over 25 up to 33% of the follicle length. Penetration beyond the infundibulum could be of crucial importance for drugs that are designed to provoke an immune response, as hair follicles are rich in immunocompetent cells in the infundibular part of the root sheath and around the excretory duct of the sebaceous gland in human hair follicles (Christoph et al., 2000).

Liposomal encapsulation of the photosensitizer 5-aminolevulinic acid (5-ALA) administered in photodynamic therapy (PDT) of *acnevulgaris* enabled a lower concentration of 5-ALA to be used, which minimizes the risk of post-treatment photosensitivity. The use of 0.5% liposome-encapsulated 5-ALA spray with intense pulsed light reduced inflammatory lesions by 52% at 1 month and 65% at 6 months after treatment of inflammatory facial acne in Asian (12 subjects), without significant side effects (Yeung et al., 2011).

Soya PC vesicles containing 1,2-dimyristoyl-sn-glycero-3-phosphocholine (DMPC) or deoxycholic acid (DA) showed increased follicular uptake of the incorporated drug chloramphenicol compared to the control solution by

1.5- and 2-fold, respectively (Hsu et al., 2017). Adapalene-loaded liposomes delivered more drug (6.72 µg/cm^2) to the hair follicles *in vitro* in pig ear skin than the gel (3.33 µg/cm^2) and drug solution (1.62 µg/cm^2). The same trend was seen regarding drug accumulation in the skin layers. CLSM images confirmed that the liposomal formulation delivered the drug into the hair follicles, which is the desired target site in the treatment of *acnevulgaris* (Kumar and Banga, 2016). Liposomal formulations loaded with three active ingredients used together against androgenic alopecia: dihomo-γ-linolenic acid, S-equol and propionyl-l-carnitine, have shown to be effective in attenuating androgenic alopecia-related hair loss in men and women, confirming the potential of liposomes to target the hair follicle (Brotzu et al., 2019).

Transfollicular drug delivery by liposomes could be used for transdermal drug delivery, especially for high molecular weight drugs, such as insulin (Kajimoto et al., 2011). The application of iontophoresis and liposomes (1,2-dioleoyl-3-(trimethylammonium) propane (DOTAP)/EPC/CHOL = 2:2:1) encapsulating insulin onto a diabetic rat skin resulted in a gradual decrease in blood glucose levels. The levels reached 20% of initial values at 18 h after administration and were maintained for up to 24 h. Hence, the authors developed an efficient non-invasive and persistent transfollicular delivery system for insulin.

Han et al. (2004) also reported enhanced transfollicular drug delivery from liposomes upon combination with iontophoresis.

2.3 NOVEL VESICLES AS TRANSDERMAL DRUG DELIVERY SYSTEMS

Nowadays it has been generally agreed that conventional liposomes are of little or no value as carriers for transdermal drug delivery, because they do not deeply penetrate the skin, but rather remain confined to the upper layers of the SC. Therefore, there was a need to develop a new generation of lipid-based vesicles. Different types of vesicles were obtained, which contain besides phospholipids and cholesterol in their bilayers, small amounts of *edge activators*, such as surfactants (e.g. polysorbate 80 (Tween® 80) or polysorbate 20 (Tween® 20)), ethanol, terpenes, etc., to enhance their membrane fluidity and deformability, i.e. elasticity, and hence their penetration-enhancing ability. Therefore these vesicles are called *elastic* or *deformable or flexible vesicles*. These elastic vesicles have shown to be superior to the conventional gel-state and even the liquid-state vesicles in terms of affecting the ultrastructure of the lipid lamellae of the SC (Van den Bergh et al., 1999a,b) as well as in terms of enhancing the drug penetration (El Maghraby et al., 1999, 2001a; Cevc and Blume, 2004; Honeywell-Nguyen et al., 2002a; Dragicevic-Curic et al., 2008). The most studied phospholipid-based elastic vesicles represent transfersomes, ethosomes, invasomes, penetration–enhancer containing vesicles, etc.

2.3.1 Transfersomes

Transfersomes® (a registered trademark of IDEA AG, Germany) represent one of the first deformable vesicles, which were introduced by Cevc (1996). These vesicles contain in their bilayers PC and edge activators (sodium cholate, polysorbate 80 or polysorbate 20), which impart deformability to the carrier, being responsible for improved transdermal drug delivery (Cevc et al., 1998, 2002, 2008a,b,c; Cevc and Blume, 2001, 2003, 2004; Cevc and Gebauer, 2003). The main benefit of using transfersomes as a carrier is the delivery of macromolecules through the skin by a non-invasive route, thereby increasing patient's compliance. They have been used for the delivery of growth hormone, insulin, proteins, vaccines, anesthetics, and herbal drugs (Gupta and Kumar, 2021). Over the past decades, the application of trans-fersomes in the field of dermal and transdermal drug delivery has been ex-tensively studied, especially as carriers for non-steroidal anti-inflammatory drugs (NSAIDs) for the treatment of inflammatory diseases. Some of the studies are described in Table 2.3.

The increased transepidermal flux profiles of drugs with Transfersomes® can be explained by the finding that the presence of a surfactant increases the elasticity of the lipid bilayers, i.e. changes the packing characteristics of the lipids in the liposome bilayers, which results in the formation of more fluid liposomes (more efficient in skin delivery of drugs), before their transfor-mation into mixed micelles (less efficient in delivery) at high surfactant concentrations (El Maghraby et al., 2004). Accordingly, it was concluded based on numerous results that flexible liposomes are more efficient in transdermal drug delivery than conventional liposomes (Table 2.3).

Ethosomes (as termed by the inventors) represent vesicles composed of phospholipids, ethanol and water. The incorporation of ethanol into lipid vesicles is an alternative approach to fluidize the lipid membrane, thereby enhancing their fluidity and elasticity, and thus improve percutaneous drug penetration (Touitou et al., 2000). Ethosomes are non-invasive delivery car-riers that enable drugs to reach the deep skin layers and/or the systemic circulation (Godin and Touitou, 2004). Thus, drugs encapsulated in etho-somes have been used in the treatment of skin diseases, hair loss,

TABLE 2.3 Examples of studies on using transfersomes as dermal and transdermal drug delivery systems

FORMULATION	DRUG	THERAPEUTIC INDICATION	EXPERIMENTAL CONDITIONS	OUTCOME	REFERENCE
Transfersomes®	Lidocaine and tetracain	Local anesthetics	*In vivo* in rats and humans	Transfersomes® provided a high local analgesic effect, which was similar to that of the corresponding s.c. injections of similar drug doses. With transfersomes the effect was higher than that of liposomes and the drug solution.	(Planas et al., 1992; Cevc, 1996)
Transfersomes® Different phospholipid: edge activator (EA) ratio	Lidocaine	Local anesthetics	In vitro	The effect of factors on vesicle size, PDI, EE% and drug release was in the rank order : lipid : EA ratio > EA type > lipid type. Optimized	(Bnyan et al., 2019)

(Continued)

TABLE 2.3 (Continued) Examples of studies on using transfersomes as dermal and transdermal drug delivery systems

FORMULATION	DRUG	THERAPEUTIC INDICATION	EXPERIMENTAL CONDITIONS	OUTCOME	REFERENCE
				transfersomes sustained the release of lidocaine over 24 h.	
Transfersomal gel with penetration enhancer (PE)-polyamidoamine dendrimer third generation (PAMAM G3)	Lidocaine	Local anesthetics	Ex vivo, permeation In vivo, tail flick test	Transfersomal gel with PE enhanced the skin permeation and local anesthetic effect of lidocaine 1,62-fold compared to the control.	(Omar et al., 2019).
Transfersomes®	TRMA, hydrocortisone and dexamethasone	Corticosteroids	In vivo, arachidonic acid-induced murine ear edema model	Transfersomes significantly increased biological potency, reduced the required drug doses (improved the therapeutic risk-benefit ratio) and enabled a sustained release	(Cevc and Blume 2003, 2004)

Transfersomes®	Dexamethasone	Corticosteroid	In vivo, carrageenan-induced rat paw edema model	in comparison to commercial preparations. Transfersomes induced better antiedema activity in comparison to liposomes and ointment. Transfersomes increased the transdermal flux, prolonged the drug release, and improved the site specificity of the drug.	(Jain Patel Madan and Lin, 2015)
Transfersomes	Diclofenac	NSAID	In vitro	Transfersomes provided a 10-fold higher drug concentration in the subcutaneous tissue compared to a commercial diclofenac gel, thus forming a drug reservoir with	(Cevc and Blume, 2001)

(Continued)

TABLE 2.3 (*Continued*) Examples of studies on using transfersomes as dermal and transdermal drug delivery systems

FORMULATION	DRUG	THERAPEUTIC INDICATION	EXPERIMENTAL CONDITIONS	OUTCOME	REFERENCE
Diractin®, transfersomal gel	Ketoprofen	NSAID	In vivo, pigs	sustained drug release. Diractin® deposited ketoprofen in deep subcutaneous tissues, which the drug from conventional gels (Gabrilen®gel, Togal® Mobil Gel, Fastum®gel) reaches mainly via systemic circulation	(Cevc et al., 2008a)
Transfersomes Different ratios of SPC:surfactants, three different surfactants (Span 20, Span 60 and Span 80).	Diclofenac	NSAID	In vitro	Transfersomes with SPC:Span 60 (2:1) were optimum vesicles regarding drug entrapment efficiency, vesicle size, zeta potential and sustained drug release.	(Shabana and Sailaja, 2015)

Transfersomes	Meloxicam	NSAID	In vitro, Shed snake skin	Transfersomes provided a significantly higher skin permeation of *meloxicam* compared to liposomes.	(Duangjit et al., 2011)
Transfersomes (SPC, sodium deoxycholate)	Celecoxib	NSAID	in-vitro and ex-vivo, drug release in-vivo, anti-inflammatory activity	Transfersomal gel was therapeutically effective in the treatment of Rheumatoid Arthritis	(Kumar, 2014)
Transfersomes (sodium deoxycholate, sodium cholate or sodium taurocholate) and ethosomes with ethanol (10, 30 or 50%) Optimum formulations were incorporated into a gel	Diflunisal	NSAID	Ex vivo, permeation In vivo, anti-inflammatory effects	Compared to the liposomal hydrogel, both hydrogels containing deformable vesicles were superior regarding diflunisal permeation and flux across the skin. They exhibited remarkable	(Abd El-Alim et al., 2019).

(Continued)

TABLE 2.3 (Continued) Examples of studies on using transfersomes as dermal and transdermal drug delivery systems

FORMULATION	DRUG	THERAPEUTIC INDICATION	EXPERIMENTAL CONDITIONS	OUTCOME	REFERENCE
				antinociceptive and anti-inflammatory effects, which was manifested by reduction in the number of writhings and higher inhibition of paw edema, indicating their use for pain and inflammation management.	
Transfersomes with Span™ 60	Colchicin	Inflammation in anti-gout therapy	In vitro and in vivo studies in rats, monosodium urate-induced air pouch model	Transfersomes encapsulating cyclodextrin-colchicine complexes enhanced skin accumulation (12.4-fold higher compared to drug solution),	(Singh et al., 2010)

				prolonged drug release and improved site specifity of colchicine.	
Core-shell gellan-transfersomes	Baicalin	Inflammatory diseases	*In vivo*, mice	Novel transfersomes improved baicalin efficacy in anti-inflammatory and skin repair tests and provided complete skin restoration.	(Manconi et al., 2018)
Tranfersomes (PC and Tween 80 or Span80) Optimized formulation was incorporated into 1% carbopol 940 gel	5-fluorouracil (5-Fu)	Antineoplastic drug for the treatment of actinic keratosis (AK) and nonmelanoma skin cancer	In vitro, permeation	The transfersomal gel showed better skin penetration and skin deposition of the drug than the marketed formulation.	(Khan et al., 2015)
Transfersomes, liposomes, and niosomes	5-fluorouracil (5-Fu)	Actinic keratosis (AK) and nonmelanoma skin cancer	In vitro, HaCaT cells, cytotoxicity	Permeation In vitro, 5-FU-loaded transfersomes were found to be most cytotoxic on the HaCaT cell line in comparison with	(Alvi et al., 2011)

(Continued)

TABLE 2.3 (Continued) Examples of studies on using transfersomes as dermal and transdermal drug delivery systems

FORMULATION	DRUG	THERAPEUTIC INDICATION	EXPERIMENTAL CONDITIONS	OUTCOME	REFERENCE
				liposomes and niosomes. We concluded that vesiculization of 5-FU not only improves the topical delivery, but also enhances the cytotoxic effect of 5-FU.	
Flexible vesicles containing Tween 20 of different surface charge	Temoporfin (mtHPC)	Fotosensitizer for PDT	In vitro, human skin	Cationic mTHPC-loaded flexible liposomes delivered the highest amount of the photosensitizer into the SC and deeper skin layers compared to conventional liposomes, neutral and anionic flexosomes	(Dragicevic-Curic et al., 2010)

Transfersomes and ethosomes	Cyclosporine A	Immunosuppresive drug for treatment of psoriasis, alopecia, etc.	in vitro	Transfersomes and ethosomes were able to effectively deliver the drug into the skin.	(Carreras et al., 2020)
Transfersomes (SPC, sodium cholate)	epigallocatechin-3-gallate (EGCG) and hyaluronic acid	Antioxidant UV radiation-protection Anti-ageing effects	In vitro, antioxidant activity ex vivo, skin permeation	Transfersomes provided significantly higher skin permeation and deposition of EGCG compared to free EGCG. They increased the cell viability and reduce lipid peroxidation, intracellular ROS levels in HaCaT cells.	(Avadhani et al., 2017).
Transfersomes (containing Tween® 20, 40, 60 or 80)	Tocopherol	Antioxidant	In vitro, permeation In vitro, in keratinocytes and fibroblasts, biocompatibility	Transfersomes have shown to bear potential as a topical delivery system with antioxidant activity and wound healing properties.	(Caddeo et al., 2018)

(Continued)

TABLE 2.3 (Continued) Examples of studies on using transfersomes as dermal and transdermal drug delivery systems

FORMULATION	DRUG	THERAPEUTIC INDICATION	EXPERIMENTAL CONDITIONS	OUTCOME	REFERENCE
Transfersomes	*Growth hormone (hGH)*	Anti-ageing	In vitro skin permeation and biological activity	They sowed biocompatibility. Encapsulated hGH increased cell migration, proliferation and collagen I and III gene expression. Transfersomes enhanced skin permeation of hGH.	(Azimi et al., 2019).
Transfersomes	Tetanus toxoid (TT)	Transcutaneous immunization	*In vivo* study, rats	TT entrapped in transfersomes, after secondary immunization, could elicit an immune response being equivalent to that produced by i.m. alum-adsorbed TT-based immunization.	(Gupta, Mishra, Singh, et al., 2005)

Transfersomes of different surface charge	DNA encoding the hepatitis B surface antigen (HBsAg)	Transcutaneous immunization	*In vivo*, mice	Cationic transfersomes loaded with HBsAg elicited a significantly higher anti-HBsAg antibody titer and cytokines level as compared to unentrapped DNA, being comparable to levels achieved after i.m. administration.	(Mahor et al., 2007).
Transfersomes (SPC, sodium cholate)	Insulin	Diabetes	*in vivo*, in mice and humans	Transfersomes enabled a systemic delivery of insulin, with efficiency comparable to that obtained after a s.c. injection of the same preparation, but with a longer lag time.	(Cevc, 1996; Cevc, 1996).
Transfersomes (SPC, Span®80)	Sertraline	Depression	In vitro, release ex vivo, permeation in vivo, modified	Transfersomal gel provided a significantly higher	(Gupta et al., 2012).

(Continued)

TABLE 2.3 (Continued) Examples of studies on using transfersomes as dermal and transdermal drug delivery systems

FORMULATION	DRUG	THERAPEUTIC INDICATION	EXPERIMENTAL CONDITIONS	OUTCOME	REFERENCE
incorporate into a carbomer gel			forced swim model test	cumulative amount of drug permeated and flux along with lower lag time than the drug solution and drug gel. Transfersomal gel had better antidepressant activity as compared to the control gel	
Transfersomes Optimum formulation was incorporated into 2% (w/v) hydroxypropyl methylcellulose hydrogel	Papaverine hydrochloride	Treatment of erectile dysfunction	In vitro In vivo	Clinical studies showed that transfersomes can be used as a carrier of papaverine hydrochloride for both diagnosis and treatment of the erectile dysfunction.	(Ali et al., 2015)

| Transfersomes(EPC, stearyl amine, Tween 20) | 19-amino-acid synthetic peptide PnPP-19 (P nigriventer potentiator peptide) | Treatment of erectile dysfunction | In vitro, human skin | Cationic transfersomes protected the peptide from degradation, and enabled a higher permeation rate, i.e., its topical administration. | (De Marco Almeida et al., 2018). |

inflammatory diseases, menopausal syndroms, transcutaneous vaccination, etc. Ethosomes loaded with a number of naturally occurring compounds for treating skin disorders as well as for cosmetic applications are also reported (Natsheh et al., 2019). Some of the studies investigating their penetration enhancing ability, as well as their therapeutic effectiveness are represented in Table 2.4.

Invasomes (as termed by the inventors) were introduced by Verma et al. (2003a). These vesicles for enhanced skin delivery of drugs contain besides PC and the aqueous phase also small amounts of ethanol and terpenes or mixtures of terpenes as penetration enhancers, which increase the fluidity of vesicle bilayers. Invasomes will be discussed in a separate chapter (chapter 3).

PEVs consist of SPC and different amounts of penetration enhancers (2-(2-ethoxyethoxy) ethanol (Transcutol®), capryl-caproyl macrogol 8-glyceride (Labrasol®), and cineole) (Mura et al., 2007, 2011). These PEVs were able to significantly improve the skin deposition of minoxidil compared to classic liposomes and solutions, without any transdermal delivery (Mura et al., 2007), as well as of other drugs. For more details refer to (Manca et al., 2016).

2.4 MECHANISMS OF ACTION OF LIPOSOMES/VESICLES

The most intriguing feature regarding liposomes is the mechanism of their penetration enhancing ability, which has not been completely clarified. Few studies have been devoted to elucidate the mechanism of the penetration-enhancing ability of vesicles. However, several mechanisms of vesicle skin interactions being responsible for the enhanced delivery of entrapped drugs have been described in the literature (Figure 2.3).

2.4.1 Penetration of Intact Liposomes/Vesicles

One of the first theories was that intact conventional liposomes could penetrate into and even through the SC (Figure 2.3) under the influence of a transepidermal osmotic gradient, acting as drug carrier systems (Cevc and Blume, 1992; Cevc et al., 2002). This theory was in accordance with the first reports on liposomes as skin delivery systems (Mezei and Gulasekharam, 1980, 1982) and with the electron micrography results revealing the presence of intact DPPC/CHOL liposomes in the dermis of guinea pigs (Foldvari et al., 1990). In addition, Egbaria et al. (1990a) found that the ratio of radiolabelled components

TABLE 2.4 Examples of studies on using ethosomes as dermal and transdermal drug delivery systems

FORMULATION	DRUG	THERAPEUTIC INDICATION	EXPERIMENTAL CONDITIONS	OUTCOME	REFERENCE
Ethosomes	Minoxidil	Hair loss	In vitro, nude mice	Ethosomes significantly enhanced in vitro the amount of minoxidil permeated through and deposited in the skin compared to ethanolic, hydroethanolic solution or the phospholipid ethanolic micellar solution of minoxidil.	(Touitou et al., 2000)
Ethosomes	Finasteride	Hair loss (Androgenetic alopecia)	In vitro, human cadaver skin	Ethosomes enhanced finasteride permeation through the skin 7.4, 3.2, 2.6-fold higher compared to liposomes, aqueous and hydroethanolic solution. Ethosomes produced a significant finasteride	(Rao et al., 2008)

(Continued)

TABLE 2.4 (Continued) Examples of studies on using ethosomes as dermal and transdermal drug delivery systems

FORMULATION	DRUG	THERAPEUTIC INDICATION	EXPERIMENTAL CONDITIONS	OUTCOME	REFERENCE
Ethosomal patch Testoderm®	Testosterone	Hypogonadal dysfunction	In vitro, rabbit pinna skin In vivo, rabbits	accumulation in the deeper skin layers. Testosterone delivery from an ethosomal patch was greater both in vitro and in vivo than from commercial patches. A 2-fold higher AUC and the highest Cmax values were obtained by ethosomal patch.	(Touitou et al., 2000)
Ethosomes	Testosterone	Hypogonadal dysfunction	In vitro, human skin In vivo, rats	Ethosomes enhanced testosterone delivery across the skin in vitro, and enabled systemic absorption of testosterone in rats.	(Ainbinder and Touitou, 2005)
Ethosomes	Trihexyphenidyl hydrochloride (THP)	Parkinson's disease	In vitro, nude mouse	The flux of THP through nude mouse skin in vitro and the quantity of the drug remaining in the skin at the end of the	(Dayan and Touitou, 2000)

Ethosomes	Acyclovir	Herpes labialis	Randomized double-blind clinical study	experiment were significantly higher when used entrapped in ethosomes compared to liposomes, phosphate buffer and the hydroethanolic solution	
				Acyclovir delivered from ethosomes performed significantly better than Zovirax®, inducing a shorter average time to crusting of lesions, shorter healing time and a higher percentage of abortive lesions.	(Horwitz et al., 1999)
Ethosomes	Acyclovir palmitate	Herpes labialis	In vitro, mice skin	Combination of the lipophilic prodrug acyclovir palmitate and ethosomes synergistically	(Zhou et al., 2010)

(Continued)

TABLE 2.4 (Continued) Examples of studies on using ethosomes as dermal and transdermal drug delivery systems

FORMULATION	DRUG	THERAPEUTIC INDICATION	EXPERIMENTAL CONDITIONS	OUTCOME	REFERENCE
				enhanced acyclovir absorption into skin.	
Ethosomes	Cannabidiol	Anti-inflammatory treatment	*In vivo*, nude mice skin	Ethosomes enhanced cannabidiol permeation through the skin and its accumulation in skin and muscle, at levels that demonstrate their potential to be used as an anti-inflammatory treatment.	(Lodzki et al., 2003)
Ethosomes	Bacitracin	Antibiotic	*In vitro, human skin In vitro, rat skin*	Bacitracin was delivered by ethosomes into the deep layers of human skin *in vitro* and rat skin *in vivo*.	(Godin and Touitou, 2004)
Ethosomes	Erythromycin	Antibiotic	*In vivo, mice*	Ethosomes delivered erythromycin to bacteria localized within the deep skin layers for eradication	(Godin and Touitou, 2005)

Ethosomes	Melatonin	Insomnia	*In vitro*, human cadaver skin	of staphylococcal infections. Ethosomes improved the transdermal delivery of melatonin, the flux was more than 2-fold higher compared to hydroethanolic solution and liposomes	(Dubey et al., 2007)
Ethosomes	Indinavir	Anti-human immunodeficiency virus (HIV) agent	In vitro	Ethosomes improved the transdermal delivery of indinavir, i.e. at least a 2 –fold higher flux was obtained as compared to hydroethanolic solution, liposomes and aqueous solution.	(Dubey et al., 2010)
Ethosomes	Buspirone hydrochloride	Treatment of menopausal syndromes	*In vitro*, porcine ear skin *In vivo*, rats	Ethosomes enhanced *in vitro* BH permeation into skin, and provided *in vivo* good bioavailability and efficient	(Shumilov and Touitou, 2010)

(*Continued*)

TABLE 2.4 (Continued) Examples of studies on using ethosomes as dermal and transdermal drug delivery systems

FORMULATION	DRUG	THERAPEUTIC INDICATION	EXPERIMENTAL CONDITIONS	OUTCOME	REFERENCE
Ethanol (3.3–20% w/v) containing vesicles	Temoporfin (mTHPC)	Fotosensitizer for PDT	In vitro, human skin	pharmacodynamic responses. Liposomes with the highest amount of ethanol delivered the highest mTHPC-amount into the SC and deeper skin layers compared to conventional liposomes, liposomes with lower ethanol amount and the ethanolic solution.	(Dragicevic-Curic et al., 2008)
Ethosomal gel	Ibuprofen	NSAID	In vivo, Brewers induced-fever in rats, and tail flick nociception in mice	Ibuprofn-ethosomal gel was present in plasma for a longer period of time as compared to the oral administration and showed a high relative bioavailability. It induced an efficient	(Shumilov et al., 2010)

Ethosomes	Diclofenac	NSAID	In vitro, permeation study In vivo, anti-inflammatory activity	antipyretic effect in fevered rats. Permeation flux for the optimized ethosomes was significantly higher than that of the drug-loaded conventional liposomes, ethanolic or aqueous solution, while the anti-inflammatory activity of ethosomal gel was higher compared to liposomal and plain gel.	(Jain et al., 2015)
Ethosomes and elastic liposomes	HBsAg	Transcutaneous vaccine against hepatitis B	In vitro uptake by human dendritic cells (DCs), and ability to stimulate T lymphocytes	HBsAg-loaded ethosomes were able to generate a protective immune response, had higher internalizing ability and immunogenicity in comparison to HBsAg-loaded elastic liposomes, which would enable	(Mishra et al., 2010)

(Continued)

TABLE 2.4 (Continued) Examples of studies on using ethosomes as dermal and transdermal drug delivery systems

FORMULATION	DRUG	THERAPEUTIC INDICATION	EXPERIMENTAL CONDITIONS	OUTCOME	REFERENCE
Optimum ethosomal formulation was incorporated into a carbomer gel (solvent: pure water or phosphate buffer saline with 30% ethanol (PBS gel))	Antigen	Vaccine delivery	In vitro, artificial membranes, release study In vitro, mice skin, permeation In vivo, immunoassay	transcutaneous vaccination against hepatitis B. Ethosomal PBS gel could deliver the antigenic molecules into the mice skin and stimulate specific IgG secretion.	(Zhang et al., 2014)
Ethosomes, liposomes, transfersomes and cubosomes	Peptide vaccine	Transcutaneous immunization	In vitro, stillborn piglet skin	Ethosomes and cubosomes induced greater peptide penetration and accumulation in the skin treated compared to liposomes and transfersomes (with these systems peptide was only located in the vicinity of the hair	(Rattanapak et al., 2012)

Ethosomes, binary ethosomes, transfersomes	Terbinafine Hydrochloride (TH)	Antimicotic drug	In vitro	follicles and within the hair shaft). Ethosomes are promising for transcutaneous immunization. Binary ethosomes most effectively enhanced drug penetration through skin; transfersomes provided drug accumulation in the skin. Ethosomes improved skin permeation more than skin deposition.	(Zhang et al., 2014)
Ethosomes	Paeonol	Anti-inflammatory, antidiabetic as well as pain-relieving activity	In vitro	Etosomes enhanced transdermal absorption and skin retention of paeonol, indicating that they could be primissing for transdermal paenol delivery.	(Ma et al., 2018)
Binary ethosomal gel	Fisetin	Skin cancer	*In vitro, rat skin* *In vivo, mice*	Ethosomal gel provided substantial increase in $C_{skin\ max}$ and AUC_{0-8}	(Moolakkadath et al., 2019)

(Continued)

TABLE 2.4 (Continued) Examples of studies on using ethosomes as dermal and transdermal drug delivery systems

FORMULATION	DRUG	THERAPEUTIC INDICATION	EXPERIMENTAL CONDITIONS	OUTCOME	REFERENCE
				in comparison to conventional gel. In vivo mice pre-treated with fisetin ethosomal gel showed marked decrease in the levels of TNF-α and IL-1α and less percentage of tumor incidences (49% and 96% respectively) as compared to the mice exposed to UV only.	
Ethosomes	Coenzyme Q10 (Q10)	Antioxidant for cutaneous disorders	Ex vivo, human skin In vitro, reconstituted human epidermis	Pretreatment with Q10 loaded-ethosomes exerted a consistent protective effect against oxidative stress, in both models, fibroblasts and in reconstituted human epidermis respectively.	(Sguizzato et al., 2020)
Ethosome and pretreatment with	5-fluorouracil	Melanoma	in vitro and in vivo, permeation study	The combination promoted significant	(Khan et al., 2015)

Drug / System	Disease	Study	Results	Reference
microwave (at 2450 MHz for 2.5 min)		In vitro, SKMEL-28 melanoma cells, cytotoxicity, uptake and intracellular trafficking	drug deposition in skin in vitro while keeping the level of drug permeation unaffected, being similar in vivo (reduced drug permeation into blood). Intracellular localization of ethosomes was enhanced.	
Paeoniflorin Ethosomes and microneedles (MNs)	Arthritis	Ex vivo, permeation	The use of ethosomes and MN can both enhance the penetration of paeoniflorin, but there was no synergism between ethosoms and MNs.	(Cui et al., 2018)

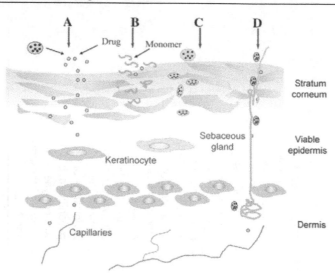

FIGURE 2.3 Mechanism of action of vesicles as skin delivery systems. (A) Free drug permeation, (B) permeation enhancement induced by liposome components, (C) penetration of intact vesicles through the SC and (D) transappendageal delivery (Zhai and Zhai, 2014).

((^{14}C) inulin and (^{3}H) CHOL) of phospholipid liposomes and SCLLs was maintained throughout the skin, indicating a carrier penetration, which was supported by a similar study with phospholipid liposomes and SCLLs (Fresta and Puglisi, 1996). This theory has been rejected by authors, who found no evidence of intact vesicles in the deeper skin layers (Lasch et al., 1991; Zellmer et al., 1995; Van Kuijk-Meuwissen et al., 1998a). However, it has been shown that liposomes can penetrate into diseased skin with a disrupted SC (as in eczema), but cannot penetrate into the skin with hyperkeratosis (as in psoriasis) (Korting et al., 1995). In diseased skin liposomes are internalized by keratinocytes via phagocitosis, being further disintegrated, thereby releasing the entrapped drug (Schaller and Korting, 1996). Lasch et al. (1991), showed by fluoromicrography that fluorescent intact PC/CHOL liposomes applied to the skin, label only the first cell layers of human SC, suggesting that intact liposomes are confined to the SC and do not penetrate deeper. However, this study could not answer the question of whether only the fluorescent markers or intact liposomes penetrated into the first SC layers. Masini et al. (1993) showed that the ratio of the labeled phospholipid and the incorporated labeled drug tretinoin was constant throughout the SC, but not in the epidermis and dermis, suggesting that liposomes could penetrate only into the SC. The results of Du Plessis et al. (1994), who did not find a higher drug deposition in the skin from smaller liposomes support the theory that intact conventional liposomes cannot penetrate through the skin. Thus, it is generally accepted that conventional liposomes do not penetrate as intact vesicles into/through the skin. As to the ultradeformable vesicles, i.e. Transfersomes®, it has been reported that these vesicles possessing high shape adaptability (i.e. ability to deform enough to fit into small pores narrower than the vesicle diameter), which depends on the bilayer flexibility due to the presence of "edge activators" (e.g. surfactants) in vesicles', and being sufficiently stable, squeeze through pores in the SC and penetrate as intact vesicles into deep subcutaneous tissue and even into systemic circulation (Cevc et al., 2008b,c) (Figure 2.4). Cevc et al. (2008b,c) proposed that Transfersomes® (as aqueos dispersion) when placed onto the skin without occlusion start to experience osmotic stress, and the "hydrational driving force" across the SC builds up (Cevc, 1996, 2002; Cevc and Blume, 1992; Schätzlein and Cevc, 1998; Cevc and Gebauer, 2003). Due to their deformability and the existing "hydrational driving force", Transfersomes® in order to avoid dry surroundings (at skin surface) and to remain maximally swollen can overcome pores much narrower than their own diameter without changing their size significantly (Cevc and Gebauer, 2003) (Figure 2.4). Hence, the drug-loaded ultradeformable vesicle is "pulled" as an intact moiety across the skin barrier along the transepidermal hydration gradient until it reaches viable epidermis where water abounds and the hydrational "pull" effect ceases (Cevc and Gebauer, 2003). However, the "pull" effect can be replaced by a "push" effect on the carriers that already crossed the barrier. Such "push" effect is exerted by the ultradeformable aggregates still sensing the hydration gradient in the dry part of the SC. Carriers consequently continue to move into the interior of the body so long as at least some of the "late-movers" remain subject to transepidermal hydration gradient.

Schätzlein and Cevc (1998) explored the intact murine SC ex vivo and in vivo by CLSM, and showed that intact deformable/elastic vesicles (Transfersomes®) after non-occlusive application penetrate into the SC through pre-existing channels, i.e. through the "intercluster" pathway – between groups of corneocytes that only partly overlap (low resistance route) with a barrier maximum at around 10 μm, being the main penetration pathway of vesicles and the "intercorneocyte" pathway – between individual corneocytes (high resistance route) with a barrier maximum at around 4–7 μm (Figure 2.5). It should be, however, stressed that CLSM cannot be used to visualize the transport of intact vesicles, but only the transport of fluorescent labels.

Van den Bergh et al. (1999b) showed in vitro in human skin using two-photon-excitation microscopy that a fluorescent label when incorporated into elastic vesicles, composed of the micelle-forming surfactant PEG-8-L (octaoxyethylene laurate ester; increasing its amount increases the bilayers' elasticity), the bilayer-forming surfactant L-595 (sucrose laurate ester) and

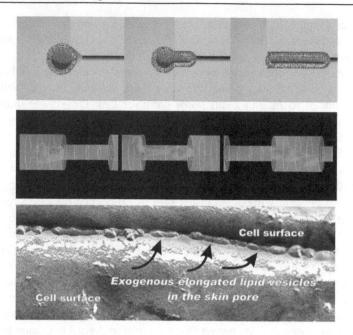

FIGURE 2.4 *Top*: computer simulated distribution of more (red, e.g. surfactant) or less (blue, e.g. a phospholipid) water soluble molecules with the hydrophobic (yellow) chains arranged in a mixed amphipats bilayer as a function of predefined vesicle shape. *Middle*: a supercomputer (CRAY) simulation of a highly deformable, infinitely permeable, non-distructible vesicle forced by a horizontal gradient ("quasi-gravitation") into a pore with 0.5 smaller diameter. *Bottom*: an electromicrograph of elongated, deformable vesicles in an inter-corneocyte hydrophilic conduit within the human stratum corneum after an application of a lipid preparation on open skin surface (Cevc and Vierl, 2010).

cholesterol sulfate (70:30:5, mol%), penetrates under non-occlusion into the SC until the SC–stratum granulosum interface through a fine meshwork of thread-like channels (Figure 2.6.), which, however, differed from the channels observed by Cevc et al. (1998). These channels were not seen after the application of rigid vesicles, micelles or the free fluorescent label. It has been shown in the same study by transmission electron microscopy (TEM) and freeze fracture electron microscopy (FFEM) that elastic vesicles (PEG-8-L:L-595, 70:30 mol%) disrupt the stacking of the lipid lamellae in the SC, thereby creating dislocations and possible penetration pathways, while rigid vesicles do not affect the ultrastructure of the skin. In contrast to the theory of intact vesicle penetration through the skin (Cevc and Blume, 1992; Cevc et al., 2008b,c), in this study intact elastic vesicles were not seen in the deepest SC

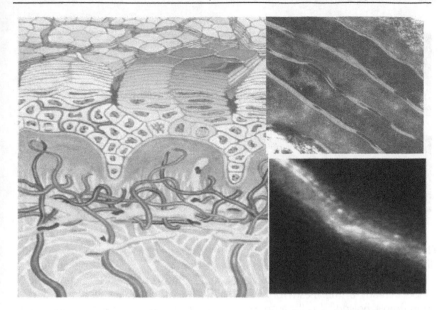

FIGURE 2.5 Schematic representation of mammalian skin, including the outer epidermis, full of tightly packed cells (corneocytes). Corneocytes are grouped in clusters, surrounded by 'furrows' or 'clefts' (with a lower permeation resistance) (left). *Upper right*: Contacts between the flat, and vertically stacked, corneocytes within the SC are sealed by inter-cellular lipids (dark lines), but water can none-theless evaporate between cells through hydrophilic conduits. *Lower right*: fluorescently labeled deformable vesicles can spontaneously widen and then tresspass the hydrophilic conduits, driven by the natural transepidermal hydration gradient, simultaneously delivering exogenous material from skin surface toward skin depth (from Cevc and Chopra, 2016, based on Cevc and Gebauer, 2003 and Schätzlein and Cevc, 1998).

layers, neither any change was observed in the ultrastructure of the viable epidermis and dermis.

Honeywell-Nguyen et al. (2002a) demonstrated *in vivo* in human skin by using FFEM the partitioning of intact elastic vesicles (L-595/PEG-8-L/sulfo-succinate (50:50:5, mol % and L-595/Tween 20/sulfosuccinate (60:40:5, mol %) into the deeper layers of the SC after their non-occlusive application. These vesicles were accumulated in channel-like regions within the intercellular lipid lamellae, which were proposed to correspond to those reported by van den Bergh et al. (1999b), having similar sizes and dimensions. Some channels were filled with fused vesicle material, but in approximately 80% of the cases, the presence of intact vesicles was demonstrated (Figure 2.7).

(a)   (b)

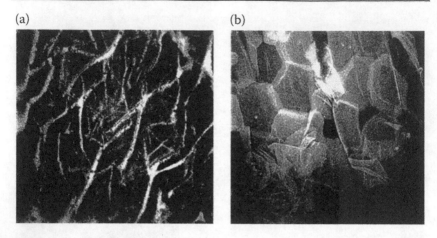

FIGURE 2.6 Two-photon excitation microscopy images of the skin treated with different vesicles (A). xy-Image recorded at a depth of 10 μm in the skin treated with PEG-8-L:L-595:CS (70:30:5, mol%) liquid-state vesicles. After 1 h of application, already a fine meshwork of "channels" was observed without any distinguishable polygonal cell contours. The distance between these channels was approximately 5 μm. (B) xy-Image recorded in the skin treated with rigid Wasag-7:CHOL:CS (50:50:5, mol%) vesicles at a depth of 3 μm in the SC. The contours of the polygonal shaped cells are clearly depicted in contrast to image of the SC obtained after treatment with elastic vesicles. CS- cholesterol sulfate, Wasag-7 consists of 70% stearate-ester and 30% palmitate-ester (40% mono, 60% di/tri-ester) (van den Bergh et al., 1999b).

Channel-like regions without vesicles were abundantly found (in tape strips 1 to 15 after tape-stripping) also in the skin treated with the buffer control, suggesting that these structures are features of normal skin. Honeywell-Nguyen et al. (2002a) proposed that intact elastic vesicles partition into the SC through pre-exisiting channels, and thereby act as "carriers" of drugs, however, *do not partition from the SC into the viable epidermis*, since only little vesicle material was found in the deepest SC layers. This was in agreement with the other findings (Van den Bergh et al., 1999b; El Maghraby et al., 1999, 2000b). As to rigid vesicles, they fused and formed lipid bilayers at the skin surface, whereas they did not induce changes in the ultrastructure of the deeper layers of the SC. An interesting finding in their investigation was that elastic vesicles in channel-like regions in the deeper SC were of smaller size than the vesicles at the skin surface, suggesting that only smaller elastic vesicles can partition into the SC through the channel-like regions (Honeywell-Nguyen et al., 2002a). However, as the distribution profiles of the incorporated drug ketorolac and elastic vesicles material were

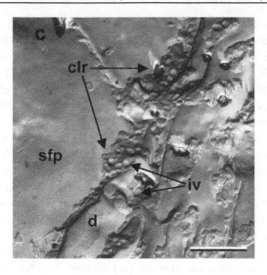

FIGURE 2.7 In vivo interactions between elastic vesicles and human skin in the deeper layers of the SC. Micrograph of the 9th tape strip of skin treated with L-595/Tween 20/sulfosuccinate (60:40:5) elastic vesicles. Channel-like regions can be seen containing vesicular structures. Fused vesicle material is also present. This strongly suggests that elastic vesicles can enter the deeper layers of the SC within 1 h of vesicle application. sfp = smooth fracture planes, d = desmosome, clr = channel-like regions, iv = intact vesicles. Scale bar represents 1 μm (Honeywell-Nguyen et al., 2002a).

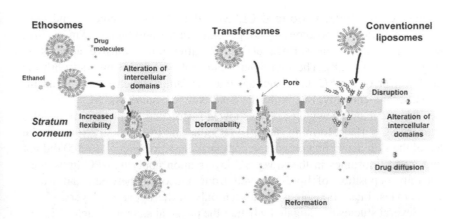

FIGURE 2.8 Proposed penetration enhancing mechanism for skin delivery of drugs from ethosomes, transfersomes and conventional liposomes (Sala et al., 2018).

different, it was suggested that once the elastic vesicles partition into the SC, the drug is released from vesicles (Honeywell-Nguyen et al., 2004).

Touitou et al. (2000) proposed a mechanism by which the flexible ethosomes could enhance drug penetration into/through skin. This mechanism involves transport pathways through the SC and the pilosebaceous units (Figure 2.8). A kind of synergistic effect of ethanol and vesicles on the skin lipids was suggested, based on the results obtained in fluorescent anisotropy and differential scanning calorimetry (DSC) measurements as well as in skin permeation studies, where it was shown that firstly ethanol disturbs the organization of the SC lipid bilayers enhancing their fluidity, and it enhances the vesicles' fluidity. Then, ethosomes can penetrate as intact vesicles the disturbed SC bilayers and even forge a pathway through the skin. The release of the drug in the deeper layers of the skin and its transdermal absorption could then be a result of the fusion of ethosomes with skin lipids and drug release at various points along the penetration pathway. Additionally, it is proposed that ethosomes are also trapped in hair follicles (Touitou et al., 2000, Ainbinder et al., 2016).

2.4.2 Penetration-Enhancing Mechanism of Vesicles' Components and Vesicle Adsorption to and/or Fusion With SC Lipids

Zellmer et al. (1995) performed CLSM and DSC measurements and concluded that DMPC liposomes do not penetrate intact into human skin *in vitro*, but disintegrate at the surface of the SC after non-occlusive application (Figures 2.3 and 2.8). The individual lipid molecules then interact with the lipid barrier of the SC and penetrate into the latter, which results in an increase of the enthalpy, related to the lipid components of the SC.

Abraham and Downing (1990) showed fusion and adsorption of vesicles onto the SC surface, forming stacks of lamellae and irregular structures on the top of the skin depending on vesicle composition. Korting et al. (1995) did not find intact liposomes in the lower SC layers upon applying SPC liposomes, but only deposition of lipids derived from liposomes between and within corneocytes. Intact liposomes were seen only in the upper SC layers.

Several studies investigated whether the physical state of vesicles (liquid-crystalline or gel state) is essential for their mode of action. Hofland et al. (1995) showed using three different liquid-state liposome formulations that two types of vesicle–skin interactions were observed *in vitro* in human skin after occlusive application: interactions at the skin–formulation interface involving adsorption and fusion of liposomes onto the outer surface of the SC, and ultrastructural changes in the deeper layers of the SC caused by mixing of the liposomal constituents and the SC lipids suggesting a penetration enhancing effect of vesicles. The main difference between the liposome formulations was the hydrophilicity and the charge of the headgroups of the main phospholipids in the commercial mixtures. Liposomes containing the largest fraction of PC, showed a marked interaction with the SC. The corneocytes were considerably swollen and the ultrastructure of the intercellular lipids showed flattened spherical structures, indicating that a high amount of vesicle lipids was dispersed in the lipid matrix of the SC. Liposomes with low PC content fused on the skin surface without inducing changes in the lipid organization of the SC. Liposomes containing lowest PC content sticked at the skin surface and rough structures up to the fourth layer of the SC were observed upon their application, which may be caused either by fusion of vesicles or by alteration of the lipid bilayer structure of the SC. These studies showed that liquid state liposomes prepared from different lipid mixtures induce different interactions with the SC.

Analogous to these liposome–skin interactions, Hofland et al. (1994) proposed two mechanisms to play an important role in nonionic surfactant vesicle–skin interactions, i.e. the penetration enhancing effect of surfactant molecules (shown by skin pre-treatment) and the effect of the vesicular structures that are most likely caused by adsorption of the vesicles at the SC–vesicle dispersion interface. Hence, a mixing of skin lipids and nonionic surfactants is proposed to occur after the application of liquid-state nonionic surfactant vesicles, while gel-state nonionic surfactant vesicles have no influence on the ultrastructure of the SC lipids and they adsorb at the SC surface. Upon applying liquid-state vesicles, there were occasionally observed vesicular structures in the deeper SC layers, and their presence was explained by the penetration of vesicle components which might be capable of reforming vesicles in the SC. In addition, water pools were formed not only in the corneocytes, but also between the corneocytes indicating a phase separation between the SC lipids and water.

Kirjavainen et al. (1996) revealed that, vesicles containing "fusogenic" cone or inverse cone shaped phospholipids, like DOPE or 1-stearoyl-sn-glycero-3-phosphocholine (stearoyl-LPC), promote the penetration of a fluorescent probe into human skin *in vitro* (shown by skin pre-treatment) in contrast to liposomes containing rod shaped phospholipids, and thereby possess penetration enhancing ability. Using CLSM, resonance energy transfer (RET) and calcein release studies it was shown that lipid components of DOPE liposomes may penetrate into the SC by adhering to the surface of the skin, and subsequently fusing and mixing with skin lipids loosening their structure. In addition, it was found that phospholipids with low transition temperature (EPC, SPC and DOPE), being at skin temperature in fluid-state, disturb the rigid structure of the SC lipid bilayers, leading to an increase in partitioning of the drug into the skin lipids, while phospholipids with high transition temperatures (in gel-state at skin temperature, 1,2-distearoyl-sn-glycero-3-phosphocholine [DSPC]) have no influence on the ultrastructure of the lipid matrix (Kirjavainen et al., 1999a). It was also concluded that penetration enhancement of drugs into the SC lipid bilayers is at least partly due to increased drug partitioning into the skin.

Van den Bergh et al. (1998) compared the mechanisms by which fluid-state DLPC vesicles and two different kinds of gel-state vesicles composed of ceramides or DSPC, interact with human SC *in vitro* under occlusion. They found that both kinds of gel-state liposomes agreggate, fuse and adhere on the SC surface, thereby depositing stacks of lamellar sheets and forming lipid bilayer networks at the SC surface. Further, for gel-state liposomes to which cholesterol sulfate was added, changes in the lipid organization in the superficial SC layers were observed. It was believed that cholesterol sulfate was responsible for the fusion of the gel-state ceramide liposomes with the intercellular lipid bilayers, which resulted in the formation of vesicular structures between the upper and lower corneocytes, as well as for the reduced cohesion between the lipid lamellae of the upper SC leading to disrupted lipid bilayers upon the application of the DSPC liposomes. Fluid-state liposomes with and without cholesterol sulfate were not able to aggregate or fuse on the SC surface, but induced deeper down in the SC changes in the intercellular lipid organization, and occasionally intracellular vesicular structures were observed in the superficial SC layers. The authors did not observe intact liposomes in the lower SC. Further, Van den Bergh et al. (1999a) showed that elastic vesicles composed of PEG-8-L and L-595 affected the ultrastructure of the SC of mice skin *in vivo* after non-occlusive application. Distinct regions with lamellar stacks derived from the vesicles were seen in the intercellular spaces of the SC *in vivo*, which disrupted their organization and led to an increased permeability of mice skin *in vitro*. In the viable epidermis no changes in the ultrastructure were observed. Treatment with rigid sucrose stearate ester (Wasag-7) vesicles did not affect the skin ultrastructure or skin permeability. Same results were obtained using human skin *in vitro* (Van den Bergh et al., 1999b), as previously described.

Yokomizo and Sagitani (1996a,b) also proposed that phospholipids as vesicle constituents act directly on the permeability barrier of the SC, since the skin pre-treatment with propylene glycol, PC or PE promoted drug permeation and shortened the lag time, in contrast to the same study on silastic membranes, and since propylene glycol, PC and PE did not significantly affect the percutaneous absorption of indomethacin through the skin missing the SC. El Maghraby et al. (1999) reported, after investigating the effect of the skin pre-treatment with non-rigid empty PC vesicles *in vitro* in human skin, a possible penetration enhancement effect of these vesicles on skin delivery of estradiol. However, comparing this enhancement with that obtained upon applying estradiol-loaded PC vesicles, being significantly higher, and realizing the importance of the preparation of phospholipids in the form of vesicles for efficient estradiol delivery, it was concluded that penetration enhancement is not the main mechanism for improved drug flux (El Maghraby et al., 2000b). The SC lipid conformational changes and percutaneous absorption of substances have been shown to be strongly correlated (Coderch et al., 1999). Coderch et al. (2000) found also a correlation between skin penetration of encapsulated substances and the fluidity of vesicles at skin temperature. This finding together with the previous one, lends support to a penetration enhancing mechanism of vesicles based on the incorporation of lipids into the intercellular domains and the modification of the fluidity of skin lipids, which can be directly related to the fluidity of the vesicles. Furthemore, the finding that the penetration enhancement of the substance was not strictly related to the encapsulation capacity would support the non-penetration of liposome structures as intact vesicles, suggesting their possible fusion with the SC lipids (Coderch et al., 2000). Fang et al. (2001a) showed that the pre-treatment with SPC liposomes and Span^{TM} 60 niosomes enhanced the permeation of enoxacin across human skin *in vitro* and its deposition in the skin, indicating that PC and Span^{TM} 60 can serve as permeation enhancers for enoxacin. Hence, liposomes and niosomes might predominantly act on the SC intercellular lipids, raising their fluidity.

2.4.3 Free Drug Process – Penetration of the Drug Released From Vesicles

One possible mechanism of drug penetration upon the application of liposomes onto the skin would be the penetration of the free drug since during the interaction of liposomes and the skin, the drug might escape from the liposomes (Figures 2.3). El Maghraby et al. (1999) found using estradiol as a model drug, that this process is of low importance, since the transdermal flux peak of estradiol appeared at a time when drug release was negligible.

2.5 CONCLUSION

Liposomes represent due to their numerous advantages promising skin delivery systems for drugs (active pharmaceutical ingredients), cosmetic actives and natural compounds. If penetration into deeper skin layers or absorption into systemic circulation is required, deformable (elastic) vesicles are recommended to be used instead of conventional liposomes.

REFERENCES

Abraham, W., Downing, D.T., 1990. Interaction between corneocytes and stratum corneum lipid liposomes in vitro. *Biochim. Biophys. Acta.* 1021, 119–125.

Agarwal, R., Katare, O.P., Vyas, S.P., 2001. Preparation and in vitro evaluation of liposomal/niosomal delivery systems for antipsoriatic drug dithranol. *Int. J. Pharm.* 228, 43–52.

Ainbinder, D., Touitou, E., 2005 Sep–Oct. Testosterone ethosomes for enhanced transdermal delivery. *Drug Deliv.* 12(5), 297–303. doi: 10.1080/10717540500176910.

Ainbinder, D., Godin, B., Touitou, E., 2016. Ethosomes: enhanced delivery of drugs to and across the skin. In: Dragicevic, N., Maibach, H. (eds.) *Percutaneous Penetration Enhancers, Chemical Methods in Penetration Enhancement, Nanocarriers.* Berlin, Heidelberg: Springer, 61–75. https://doi.org/10.1007/978-3-662-47862-2_4

Akbarzadeh, A., Rezaei-Sadabady, R., Davaran, S., et al., 2013. Liposome: classification, preparation, and applications. *Nanoscale Res. Lett.* 8(1), 102.

Ali, M.F.M. *et al.*, 2015. Preparation and clinical evaluation of nano-transferosomes for treatment of erectile dysfunction. *Drug Des. Devel. Ther.* 9, pp. 2431–2447. doi: 10.2147/DDDT.S81236.

Alvi, I.A., Madan, J., Kaushik, D., Sardana, S., Pandey, R.S., Ali, A., 2011 Sep. Comparative study of transfersomes, liposomes, and niosomes for topical delivery of 5-fluorouracil to skin cancer cells: preparation, characterization, invitro release, and cytotoxicity analysis. *Anticancer Drugs.* 22(8), 774–782. doi: 10.1097/CAD.0b013e328346c7d6.

Ascenso, A., Raposo S., Batista C., Cardoso P., Mendes T., Praça F.G., Bentley M.V.L.B., Simões S., 2015. Development, characterization, and skin delivery studies of related ultradeformable vesicles: transfersomes, ethosomes, and transethosomes. *Int. J. Nanomed.* 10, 5837–5851.

Augustin, M., Goepel, L., Jacobi, A., Bosse, B., Mueller, S., Hopp, M., 2017. Efficacy and tolerability of liposomal polyvinylpyrrolidone-iodine hydrogel for the localized treatment of chronic infective, inflammatory, dermatoses: an uncontrolled pilot study. *Clin. Cosmet. Investig. Dermatol.* 10, 373–384.

Avadhani, K.S., Manikkath, J., Tiwari, M., Chandrasekhar, M., Godavarthi, A., Vidya, S.M., Hariharapura, R.C., Kalthur, G., Udupa, N., Mutalik, S., 2017. Skin delivery of epigallocatechin-3-gallate (EGCG) and hyaluronic acid loaded nano-transfersomes for antioxidant and anti-aging effects in UV radiation induced skin damage. *Drug Deliv.* 24(1), 61–74.

Azimi, M. *et al.*, 2019. Impact of the transfersome delivered human growth hormone on the dermal fibroblast cells. *Curr. Pharm. Biotechnol.* 20, 1194–1202.

Bangham, A.D., Horne, R.W., 1964. Negative staining of phospholipids and their structural modification by surface active agents as observed in the electron microscope. *J. Mol. Biol.* 8, 660–668.

Bangham, A.D., Standish, M.M., Watkins, J.C., 1965. Diffusion of univalent ions across the lamellae of swollen phospholipids. *J. Mol. Biol.* 13, 238–252.

Belhaj, N., Arab-Tehrany E., Loing E., Bézivin C. 2017. Skin delivery of hydrophilic molecules from liposomes and polysaccharide-coated liposomes. *Int. J. Cosmet. Sci.* 39(4), 435–441.

Bennett, W.F., MacCallum, J.L., Tieleman, D.P., 2009. Thermodynamic analysis of the effect of cholesterol on dipalmitoylphosphatidylcholine lipid membranes. *J. Am. Chem. Soc.* 131(5), 1972–1978.

Betz, G., Imboden, R., Imanidis, G., 2001. Interaction of liposome formulations with skin in vitro. *Int. J. Pharm.* 229, 117–129.

Bhatia, A., Kumar, R., Katare, O.P., 2004. Tamoxifen in topical liposomes: development, characterization and in-vitro evaluation. *J. Pharm. Pharm. Sci.* 7(2), 252–259.

Bhatia, E., Sharma, S., Jadhav, K., Banerjee, R., 2021. Combinatorial liposomes of berberine and curcumin inhibit biofilm formation and intracellular methicillin resistant *Staphylococcus aureus* infections and associated inflammation. *J. Mater. Chem. B* 9(3), 864–875.

Bhatia, A., Goni, V., Chopra, S., Singh, B., Katare, O.P., 2020. Evaluation of efficacy and safety of a novel lipogel containing diclofenac: a randomized, placebo controlled, double-blind clinical trial in patients with signs and symptoms of osteoarthritis. *Contemp. Clin. Trials Commun.* 20, 100664.

Bnyan, R., Khan, I., Ehtezazi, T., Saleem, I., Gordon, S., O'Neill F., Roberts, M., 2019. Formulation and optimisation of novel transfersomes for sustained release of local anaesthetic. *J. Pharm. Pharmacol.* 71(10), 1508–1519.

Brotzu, G., Fadda, A.M., Manca, M.L., Manca, T., Marongiu, F., Campisi, M., Consolaro, F., 2019. A liposome-based formulation containing equol, dihomo-γ-linolenic acid and propionyl-l-carnitine to prevent and treat hair loss: a prospective investigation. *Dermatol. Ther.* 32(1), e12778.

Burnette, R.R., Ongpipattanakul, B., 1987. Characterization of the permselective properties of excised human skin during iontophoresis. *J. Pharm. Sci.* 76, 765–773.

Caddeo, C., Nacher A., Vassallo A., Armentano M.F., Pons R., Fernàndez-Busquets X., Carbone C., Valenti D., Fadda A.M., Manconi M., 2016. Effect of quercetin and resveratrol co-incorporated in liposomes against inflammatory/oxidative response associated with skin cancer. *Int. J. Pharm.* 513(1–2):153–163. doi: 10.1016/j.ijpharm.2016.09.014

Campani, V., Scotti, L., Silvestri, T., Biondi, M., De Rosa, G., 2020. Skin permeation and thermodynamic features of curcumin-loaded liposomes. *J. Mater. Sci. Mater. Med.* 31(2), 18.

Carreras, J.J. *et al.*, 2020. Ultraflexible lipid vesicles allow topical absorption of cyclosporin A. *Drug Deliv. Trans. Res.* 10(2), pp. 486–497. doi: 10.1007/s13346-019-00693-4.

Castañeda-Reyes, E.D., Perea-Flores, M.J., Davila-Ortiz, G., Lee, Y., Gonzalez de Mejia, E., 2020. Development, characterization and use of liposomes as amphipathic transporters of bioactive compounds for melanoma treatment and reduction of skin inflammation: a review. *Int. J. Nanomed.* 15, 7627–7650.

Castro, G.A., Ferreira, L.A., 2008. Novel vesicular and particulate drug delivery systems for topical treatment of acne. *Expert Opin. Drug Deliv.* 5, 665–679.

Cevc, G., 1996. Transfersomes, liposomes and other lipid suspensions on the skin: permeation enhancement, vesicle penetration, and transdermal drug delivery. *Crit. Rev. Ther. Drug Carrier Syst.* 13, 257–388.

Cevc, G., 2002. Transfersomes-innovative transdermal drug carriers. In: Rathbone, M., Hadgraft, J. (eds.) *Modified Release Drug Technology.* New York: Marcel Dekker, 533–546.

Cevc, G., Blume, G., 2001. New, highly efficient formulation of diclofenac for the topical, transdermal administration in ultradeformable drug carriers. *Transfersomes. Biochim. Biophys. Acta.* 1514, 191–205.

Cevc, G. *et al.*, 1998. Ultraflexible vesicles, transfersomes, have an extremely low pore penetration resistance and transport therapeutic amounts of insulin across the intact mammalian skin. *Biochimica et Biophysica Acta – Biomembranes* 1368(2), 201–215. doi: 10.1016/S0005-2736(97)00177-6.

Cevc, G., Chopra, A., 2016. Deformable (transfersome®) vesicles for improved drug delivery into and through the skin. In: Dragicevic, N., Maibach, H. (eds.) *Percutaneous Penetration Enhancers, Chemical Methods in Penetration Enhancement, Nanocarriers.* Berlin, Heidelberg: Springer, 39–59. https://doi.org/10.1007/978-3-662-47862-2_3

Cevc, G., Blume, G., 1992. Lipid vesicles penetrate into intact skin owing to the transdermal osmotic gradients and hydration force. *Biochim. Biophys. Acta* 1104, 226–232.

Cevc, G., Gebauer, D., 2003. Hydration-driven transport of deformable lipid vesicles through fine pores and skin barrier. *Biophys. J.* 84, 1010–1024.

Cevc, G., Blume, G., 2004. Hydrocortisone and dexamethasone in very deformable drug carriers have increased biological potency, prolonged effect, and reduced therapeutic dosage. *Biochim. Biophys. Acta* 1663, 61–73

Cevc, G., Schätzlein, A., Blume, G., 1995. Transdermal drug carriers: basic properties, optimization and transfer efficiency in the case of epicutaneously applied peptides. *J. Controlled Release* 36(1–2), 3–16. doi: 10.1016/0168-3659(95)00056-E.

Cevc, G., Schätzlein, A., Richardsen, H., 2002. Ultradeformable lipid vesicles can penetrate skin and other semi-permeable membrane barriers unfragmented. Evidence from double label CLSM experiments and direct size measurement. *Biochim. Biophys. Acta* 1564, 21–30.

Cevc, G., Mazgareanu, S., Rother, M., 2008b. Preclinical characterisation of NSAIDs in ultradeformable carriers or conventional topical gels. *Int. J. Pharm.* 360, 29–39.

Cevc, G., Vierl, U., Mazgareanu, S., 2008a. Functional characterisation of novel analgesic product based on self-regulating drug carriers. *Int. J. Pharm.* 360, 18–28.

Cevc, G., Vierl, U., 2010. Nanotechnology and the transdermal route: a state of the art review and critical appraisal. *J Control Release.* 141(3), 277–299. doi: 10.1016/j.jconrel.2009.10.016.

Cevc, G., Mazgareanu, S., Rother, M., Vierl, U., 2008c. Occlusion effect on transcutaneous NSAID delivery fromconventional and carrier-based formulations. *Int. J. Pharm.* 359, 190–197.

Christoph, T., Müller-Röver, S., Audring, H., Tobin, D.J., Hermes, B., Cotsarelis, G., Rückert, R., Paus, R., 2000. The human hair follicle immune system: cellular composition and immune privilege. *Br. J. Dermatol.* 142, 862–873.

Coderch, L., de Pera, M., Perez-Cullell, N., Estelrich, J., de la Maza, A., Parra, J.L., 1999. The effect of liposomes on skin barrier structure. *Skin Pharmacol. Appl. Skin Physiol.* 12, 235–246.

Coderch, L., Fonollosa, J., De Pera, M., Estelrich, J., De La Maza, A., Para, J.L., 2000. Influence of cholesterol on liposome fluidity by EPR relationship with percutaneous absorption. *J. Control. Release.* 68, 85–95.

Cui, Y., Mo Y., Zhang, Q., Tian, W., Xue, Y., Bai, J., Du, S., 2018 Dec 19. Microneedle-assisted percutaneous delivery of paeoniflorin-loaded ethosomes. *Molecules* 23(12), 3371. doi: 10.3390/molecules23123371.

Dayan, N., Touitou, E., 2000. Carriers for skin delivery of trihexyphenidyl HCl: ethosomes vs. liposomes. *Biomaterials.* 21, 1879–1885.

de Leeuw, J., de Vijlder, H.C., Bjerring, P., Neumann, H.A., 2009. Liposomes in dermatology today. *J. Eur. Acad. Dermatol. Venereol.* 23, 505–516. doi: 10.1111/j.1468-3083.2009.03100.x.

De Marco Almeida, F. *et al.*, 2018. Physicochemical Characterization and Skin Permeation of Cationic Transfersomes Containing the Synthetic Peptide PnPP-19. *Curr. Drug Deliv.* 15(7), pp. 1064–1071. doi: 10.2174/1567201815666618010 08170206.

Doppalapudi, S., Jain, A., Chopra, D.K., Khan, W., 2017. Psoralen loaded liposomal nanocarriers for improved skin penetration and efficacy of topical PUVA in psoriasis. *Eur. J. Pharm. Sci.* 96, 515–529.

Dowton, S.M., Hu, Z., Ramachandran, C., Wallach, D.F.H., Weiner, N., 1993. Influence of liposomal composition on topical delivery of encapsulated cyclosporine A. I. An in vitro study using hairless mouse skin. *STP Pharm. Sci.* 3, 404–407.

Dragicevic-Curic, N., Scheglmann, D., Albrecht, V., Fahr, A., 2008. Temoporfin-loaded invasomes: development, characterization and in vitro skin penetration studies. *J. Control Release.* 127(1), 59–69.

Dragicevic-Curic, N., Scheglmann, D., Albrecht, V., Fahr, A., 2009. Development of liposomes containing ethanol for skin delivery of temoporfin: characterization and in vitro penetration studies. *Colloids Surf B Biointerfaces.* 74(1), 114–122. doi: 10.1016/j.colsurfb.2009.07.005.

Dragicevic-Curic, N., Gräfe, S., Gitter, B., Winter, S., Fahr, A., 2010. Surface charged temoporfin-loaded flexible vesicles: in vitro skin penetration studies and stability. *Int. J. Pharm.* 384(1–2), 100–108.

Dragicevic-Curic, N., Friedrich, M., Petersen, S., Scheglmann, D., Douroumis, D., Plass, W., Fahr, A., 2011. Assessment of fluidity of different invasomes by electron spin resonance and differential scanning calorimetry. *Int. J. Pharm.* 412(1-2), 85–94.

Du Plessis, J., Egbaria, K., Ramachandran, C., Weiner, N.D., 1992. Topical delivery of liposomally encapsulated gamma-interferon. *Antiviral Res.* 18, 259–265.

Du Plessis, J., Ramachandran, C., Weiner, N., Muller, D.G., 1994. The influence of particle size of liposomes on the disposition of drug into skin. *Int. J. Pharm.* 103, 277–282.

Duangjit, S., Opanasopit, P., Rojanarata, T., Ngawhirunpat, T., 2011. Characterization and in vitro skin permeation of meloxicam-loaded liposomes versus transfersomes. *J. Drug Deliv.* 2011, 418316. doi: 10.1155/2011/418316. Epub 2010 Nov 7. PMID: 21490750; PMCID: PMC3066552.

Dubey, V., Mishra, D., Jain, N.K., 2007. Melatonin loaded ethanolic liposomes: physicochemical characterization and enhanced transdermal delivery. *Eur. J. Pharm. Biopharm.* 67(2), 398–405. doi: 10.1016/j.ejpb.2007.03.007.

Dubey V., Mishra D., Nahar M., Jain V., Jain N.K., 2010. Enhanced transdermal delivery of an anti-HIV agent via ethanolic liposomes. *Nanomedicine* 6(4), 590–596. doi: 10.1016/j.nano.2010.01.002.

Egbaria, K., Ramachandran, C., Weiner, N., 1990b. Topical delivery of ciclosporin: evaluation of various formulations using in vitro diffusion studies in hairless mouse skin. *Skin Pharmacol.* 3, 21–28.

Egbaria, K., Ramachandran, C., Kittayanond, D., Weiner, N., 1990a. Topical delivery of liposomally encapsulated interferon evaluated by in vitro diffusion studies. *Antimicrob. Agents Chemother.* 34, 107–110

El Maghraby, G.M., Williams, A.C., 2009. Vesicular systems for delivering conventional small organic molecules and larger macromolecules to and through human skin. *Expert Opin. Drug Deliv.* 6, 149–163.

El Maghraby, G.M., Williams, A.C., Barry, B.W., 1999. Skin delivery of oestradiol from deformable and traditional liposomes: mechanistic studies. *J. Pharm. Pharmacol.* 51, 1123–1134.

El Maghraby, G.M., Williams, A.C., Barry, B.W., 2000a. Oestradiol skin delivery from ultradeformable liposomes: refinement of surfactant concentration. *Int. J. Pharm.* 196, 63–74.

El Maghraby, G.M., Williams, A.C., Barry, B.W., 2000b. Skin delivery of oestradiol from lipid vesicles: importance of liposome structure. *Int. J. Pharm.* 204, 159–169.

El Maghraby, G.M., Williams, A.C., Barry, B.W., 2001a. Skin delivery of 5-fluorouracil from ultradeformable and standard liposomes in vitro. *J. Pharm. Pharmacol.* 53, 1069–1077.

El Maghraby, G.M., Williams, A.C., Barry, B.W., 2001b. Skin hydration and possible shunt route penetration in controlled skin delivery of estradiol from ultradeformable and standard liposomes in vitro. *J. Pharm. Pharmacol.* 53, 1311–1322.

El Maghraby, G.M., Williams, A.C., Barry, B.W., 2004. Interactions of surfactants (edge activators) and skin penetration enhancers with liposomes. *Int. J. Pharm.* 276, 143–161.

El Maghraby, G.M., Barry, B.W., Williams, A.C., 2008. Liposomes and skin: from drug delivery to model membranes. *Eur. J. Pharm. Sci.* 34, 203–222.

El-Alim, A., Hosam, S., Kassem, A.A., Basha, M., Salama, A., 2019. Comparative study of liposomes, ethosomes and transfersomes as carriers for enhancing the transdermal delivery of diflunisal: in vitro and in vivo evaluation. *Int. J. Pharm.* 563, 293–303.

Elsabahy, M., Foldvari, M., 2013a. Needle-free gene delivery through the skin: an overview of recent strategies, *Curr. Pharm. Des.*, 19(41), 7301–7315.

Erdogan, M., Wright, J.R., McAlister, V.C., 2002. Liposomal tacrolimus lotion as a novel topical agent for treatment of immune-mediated skin disorders: experimental studies in a murine model. *Br. J. Dermatol.* 146, 964–967.

Esposito, E., Zanella, C., Cortesi, R., Menegatti, E., Nastruzzi, C., 1998. Influence of liposomal formulation parameters on the in vitro absorption of methyl nicotinate. *Int. J. Pharm.* 172, 255–260.

Fang, J.Y., Hong, C.T., Chiu, W.T., Wang, Y.Y., 2001a. Effect of liposomes and niosomes on skin permeation of enoxacin. *Int. J. Pharm.* 219, 61–72.

Fathalla, D., Youssef, E.M.K., Soliman, G.M., 2020. Liposomal and ethosomal gels for the topical delivery of anthralin: preparation, comparative evaluation and clinical assessment in psoriatic patients. *Pharmaceutics* 12(5), 446.

Foldvari, M., Gesztes, A., Mezei, M., 1990. Dermal drug delivery by liposome encapsulation: clinical and electron microscopic studies. *J. Microencapsul.* 7, 479–489.

Fresta, M., Puglisi, G., 1996. Application of liposomes as potential cutaneous drug delivery systems. In vitro and in vivo investigation with radioactivity labelled vesicles. *J. Drug Target.* 4, 95–101.

Gabrijelcic, V., Sentjurc, M., Schara, M., 1994. The measurement of liposome entrapped molecules' penetration into the skin: A 1D-EPR and EPR kinetic imaging study. *Int. J. Pharm.* 102, 151–158.

Gesztes, A., Mezei, M., 1988. Topical anaesthesia of skin by liposome-encapsulated tetracaine. *Anesth. Analg.* 67, 1079–1081.

Ghanbarzadeh, S., Arami, S., 2013. Enhanced transdermal delivery of diclofenac sodium via conventional liposomes, ethosomes, and transfersomes. *Biomed. Res. Int.* 1–7.

Godin, B., Touitou, E., 2004 Feb 10. Mechanism of bacitracin permeation enhancement through the skin and cellular membranes from an ethosomal carrier. *J. Control Release.* 94(2-3), 365–379. doi: 10.1016/j.jconrel.2003.10.014.

Godin, B., Touitou, E., 2005 Jul. Erythromycin ethosomal systems: physicochemical characterization and enhanced antibacterial activity. *Curr. Drug Deliv.* 2(3), 269–275. doi: 10.2174/1567201054367931.

Gupta, A. *et al.*, 2012. Transfersomes: a novel vesicular carrier for enhanced transdermal delivery of sertraline: development, characterization, and performance evaluation. *Sci. Pharm. Sci Pharm.* 80(4), 1061–1080. doi: 10.3797/scipharm.12 08-02.

Gupta, R., Kumar, A., 2021. Transfersomes: the ultra-deformable carrier system for non-invasive delivery of drug. *Curr. Drug Deliv.* 18(4), 408–420. doi: 10.2174/15 67201817666200804105416

Gupta, P.N., Mishra, V., Singh, P., *et al.*, 2005. Tetanus toxoid-loaded transfersomes for topical immunization. *J. Pharm. Pharmacol.* 57(3), pp. 295–301. doi: 10.1211/ 0022357055515.

Han, I., Kim, M., Kim, J., 2004. Enhanced transfollicular delivery of adriamycin with a liposome and iontophoresis. *Exp. Dermatol.* 13, 86–92.

Hasanovic, A., Hollick, C., Fischinger, K., Valenta, C., 2010. Improvement in physicochemical parameters of DPPC liposomes and increase in skin permeation of aciclovir and minoxidil by the addition of cationic polymers. *Eur. J. Pharm. Biopharm.* 75, 148–153.

Hoffman, R.M., 2005. Gene and stem cell therapy of the hair follicle. *Methods Mol. Biol.* 289:437–448.

Hofland, H.E.J., Geest, R., Bodde, H.E., Junginger, H.E., Bouwstra, J.A., 1994. Estradiol permeation from nonionic surfactant vesicles through human stratum corneum in vitro. *Pharm. Res.* 5, 78–89.

Hofland, H.E.J., Bouwstra, J.A., Bodde, H.E., Spies, F., Junginger, H.E., 1995. Interactions between liposomes and human stratum corneum in vitro: freeze fracture electron microscopical visualization and small angle X-ray scattering studies. *Br. J. Dermatol.* 132, 853–865.

Honeywell-Nguyen, P.L., Gooris, G.S., Bouwstra, J.A., 2004. Quantitative assessment of the transport of elastic and rigid vesicle components and a model drug from these vesicle formulations into human skin in vivo. *J. Invest. Dermatol.* 123, 902–910.

Honeywell-Nguyen, P.L., De Graaff, A.M., Wouter Groenink, H.W., Bouwstra, J.A., 2002a. The in vivo and in vitro interactions of elastic and rigid vesicles with human skin. *Biochim. Biophys. Acta* 1573, 130–140.

Horwitz, E., Pisanty, S., Czerninski, R., Helser, M., Eliav, E., Touitou, E., 1999 Jun. A clinical evaluation of a novel liposomal carrier for acyclovir in the topical treatment of recurrent herpes labialis. *Oral Surg. Oral Med. Oral Pathol. Oral Radiol. Endod.* 87(6), 700–705. doi: 10.1016/s1079-2104(99)70164-2.

Hsu, C.Y., Yang, S.C., Sung, C.T., Weng, Y.H., Fang, J.Y., 2017. Anti-MRSA malleable liposomes carrying chloramphenicol for ameliorating hair follicle targeting. *Int. J. Nanomed.* 12, 8227–8238.

Hussain, A., Altamimi M.A., Alshehri S., Imam S.S., Singh S.K., 2020. Vesicular elastic liposomes for transdermal delivery of rifampicin: in-vitro, in-vivo and in silico gastroplus^{TM} prediction studies. *Eur. J. Pharm. Sci.* 151, 105411. doi: 10.1016/j.ejps.2020.105411. Epub 2020 Jun 4. PMID: 32505794.

Jaafari, M.R., Hatamipour, M., Alavizadeh, S.H., Abbasi, A., Saberi, Z., Rafati, S., Taslimi, Y., Mohammadi, A.M., Khamesipour, A., 2019. Development of a topical liposomal formulation of Amphotericin B for the treatment of cutaneous leishmaniasis. *Int J Parasitol Drugs Drug Resist.* 11, 156–165. doi: 10.1016/ j.ijpddr.2019.09.004

Jain, S. *et al.*, 2003. Transfersomes – a novel vesicular carrier for enhanced transdermal delivery: development, characterization, and performance evaluation. *Drug Develop. Ind. Pharm.* 29(9), 1013–1026. doi: 10.1081/DDC-120025458.

Jain, S., Patel, N., Madan, P., Lin, S., 2015. Quality by design approach for formulation, evaluation and statistical optimization of diclofenac-loaded ethosomes via transdermal route. *Pharm. Dev. Technol.* 20(4), 473–489.

Jain, S., Patel, N., Madan, P., Lin, S., 2015. Quality by design approach for formulation, evaluation and statistical optimization of diclofenac-loaded ethosomes via transdermal route. *Pharm. Dev. Technol.* 20(4), 473–489.

Jeon, S., Yoo, C.Y., Park, S.N., 2015. Improved stability and skin permeability of sodium hyaluronate-chitosan multilayered liposomes by Layer-by-Layer electrostatic deposition for quercetin delivery. *Colloids Surf. B Biointerfaces.* 129, 7–14.

Jeong, S., Lee J., Im B.N., Park H., Na K., 2017. Combined photodynamic and antibiotic therapy for skin disorder via lipase-sensitive liposomes with enhanced antimicrobial performance. *Biomaterials* 141(October), 243–250.

Joseph, J., Vedha Hari B.N., Devi D.R., 2018. Experimental optimization of lornoxicam liposomes for sustained topical delivery. *Eur. J. Pharm. Sci.* 112, 38–51.

Jung, S., Otberg, N., Thiede, G., Richter, H., Sterry, W., Panzner, S., Lademann, J., 2006. Innovative liposomes as a transfollicular drug delivery system: penetration into porcine hair follicles. *J. Invest. Dermatol.* 126, 1728–1732.

Kajimoto, K., Yamamoto M., Watanabe M., Kigasawa K., Kanamura K., Harashima H., Kogure K., 2011. Noninvasive and persistent transfollicular drug delivery system using a combination of liposomes and iontophoresis. *Int. J. Pharm.* 403(1–2), 57–65.

Katahira, N., Murakami, T., Kugai, S., Yata, N., Takano, M., 1999. Enhancement of topical delivery of a lipophilic drug from charged multilamellar liposomes. *J. Drug Target.* 6, 405–414.

Khan, N.R., Wong, T.W., 2018. 5-Fluorouracil ethosomes – skin deposition and melanoma permeation synergism with microwave. *Artif. Cells Nanomed. Biotechnol.* 46(Suppl 1), 568–577. doi: 10.1080/21691401.2018.1431650.

Khan, M.A., Pandit, J., Sultana, Y., et al., 2015. Novel carbopolbased transfersomal gel of 5-fluorouracil for skin cancer treatment: in vitro characterization and in vivo study. *Drug Deliv.* 22, 795–802

Kim, M.K., Chung, S.J., Lee, M.H., Cho, A.R., Shim, C.K., 1997. Targeted and sustained delivery of hydrocortisone to normal and stratum corneum-removed skin without enhanced skin absorption using a liposome gel. *J. Control. Release* 46, 243–251.

Kinsky, S.C., Haxby, J., Kinsky, C.B., Demel, R.A., van Deenen, L.L.M., 1968. Effect of cholesterol incorporation on the sensitivity liposomes to the polyene antibiotic, filipin. *Biochim. Biophys. Acta* 152(1), 174–185.

Kirjavainen, M., Urtti, A., Valjakka-Koskela, R., Kiesvaara, J., Mönkkönen, J., 1999b. Liposome – skin interactions and their effects on the skin permeation of drugs. *Eur. J. Pharm. Sci.* 7, 279–286.

Kirjavainen, B.M., Mönkkönen, J., Saukkosaari, M., Valjakka-Koskela, R., Kiesvaara, J., Urtti, A., 1999a. Phospholipids affect stratum corneum lipid bilayer fluidity and drug partitioning into the bilayers. *J. Control. Release.* 58, 207–214.

Kirjavainen, M., Urti, A., Jääskeläinen, L., Suhonen, T.M., Paronen, P., Valjakka-Koskela, R., Kiesvaara, J., Mönkkönen, J., 1996. Interaction of liposomes with human skin in vitro–the influence of lipid composition and structure. *Biochim. Biophys. Acta* 1304, 179–189.

102   Invasomes as Drug Nanocarriers

Knepp, V.M., Szoka, F.C., Guy, R.H., 1990. Controlled drug release from a novel liposome delivery system. II. Transdermal delivery characteristics. *J. Control. Release* 12, 25–30.

Knepp, V.M., Hinz, R.S., Szoka, F.C., Guy, R.H., 1988. Controlled drug release from a novel liposomal delivery system. I. Investigations of transdermal potential. *J. Control. Release* 5, 211–221.

Korting, H.C., Stolz, W., Schmid, M.H., Maierhofer, G., 1995. Interaction of liposomes with human epidermis reconstructed in vitro. *Br. J. Dermatol.* 132, 571–579.

Kriftner, R.W., 1992. Liposome Production: The Ethanol injection Technique and the Development of the First Approved Liposome Dermatic. In: Braun-Falco, O., Korting, H.C., Maibach, H.I. (Eds.), *Liposome Dermatics.* Springer-Verlag, Berlin, pp. 91–100.

Kumar, M.S., Preeti, 2014. Development of celecoxibtransfersomal gel for the treatment of rheumatoid arthritis. *Indian J. Pharm. Boil. Res.* 2, 7–13.

Kumar, V., Banga, A.K., 2016. Intradermal and follicular delivery of adapalene liposomes. *Drug Dev. Ind. Pharm.* 42(6), 871–879.

Lasch, J., Laub, R., Wohlrab, W., 1991. How deep do intact liposomes penetrate into human skin? *J. Control. Release* 18, 55–58.

Lauer, A.C., 1999. Percutaneous drug delivery to the hair follicle. Third edition. In: Bronaugh R.L., Maibach H.I. (eds) *Percutaneous Absorption Drugs-Cosmetics-Mechanisms-Methodology.* Marcel Dekker, Inc., New York, Basel, pp. 427–449.

Lautenschläger, H., 2006. Liposomes. In: Barel A.O., Paye M., Maibach H.I., (eds) *Handbook of Cosmetic Science and Technology.* CRC Press Taylor & Francis Group, Boca Raton, pp. 155–163.

Li, L., Hoffman, R.M., 1997. Topical liposome delivery of molecules to hair follicles in mice. *J. Derm. Sci.* 14, 101–108.

Li, L., Margolis, L.B., Lishko, L.V., 1992. Product-delivering liposomes specifically target entrapped melanin to hair follicles in histocultured intact skin. *In Vitro Cell. Dev. Biol.* 28A, 679–681.

Li, L., Lishko, L.V., Hoffman, R.M., 1993a. Liposomes can specifically target entrapped melanin to hair follicles in histocultured skin. *In Vitro Cell. Dev. Biol.* 29A, 192–194.

Li, L., Lishko, L.V., Hoffman, R.M., 1993b. Liposomes targeting high molecular weight DNA to hair follicles in histocultured skin: a model for gene therapy of the hair growth process. *In Vitro Cell. Dev. Biol.* 29A, 258–260.

Li, Z., Liu, M., Wang, H., Du, S., 2016. Increased cutaneous wound healing efect of biodegradable liposomes containing madecassoside: preparation optimization, in vitro dermal permeation, and in vivo bioevaluation. *Int. J. Nanomed.* 11:2995–3007.

Lieb, L.M., Flynn, G., Weiner, N., 1994. Follicular (pilosebaceous unit) deposition and pharmacological behavior of cimetidine as a function of formulation. *Pharm. Res.* 11, 1419–1423.

Lieb, L.M., Ramachandran, C., Egbaria, K., Weiner, N., 1992. Topical delivery enhancement with multilamellar liposomes into pilosebaceous units. I. In vitro evaluation using fluorescent techniques with hamster ear model. *J. Invest. Dermatol.* 99, 108–113.

Lin, M.W., Huang, Y.B., Chen, C.L., Wu, P.C., Chou, C.Y., Wu, P.C., Hung, S.Y., 2016. A formulation study of 5-aminolevulinic encapsulated in DPPC liposomes in melanoma treatment. *Int. J. Med. Sci.* 13(7), 483–489.

Liu, H., Pan, W.S., Tang, R., Luo, S.D., 2004. Topical delivery of different acyclovir palmitate liposome formulations through rat skin in vitro. *Pharmazie* 59, 203–206.

Lodzki, M., Godin, B., Rakou, L., Mechoulam, R., Gallily, R., Touitou, E., 2003 Dec 12. Cannabidiol-transdermal delivery and anti-inflammatory effect in a murine model. *J Control Release.* 93(3), 377–387. doi: 10.1016/j.jconrel.2003.09.001.

Ma, H., Guo, D., Fan, Y., Wang, J., Cheng, J., Zhang, X., 2018 Jul 17. Paeonol-loaded ethosomes as transdermal delivery carriers: design, preparation and evaluation. *Molecules* 23(7), 1756. doi: 10.3390/molecules23071756.

Mahor, S. *et al.*, 2007. Cationic transfersomes based topical genetic vaccine against hepatitis B. *Int. J. Pharm.* 340(1–2), 13–19. doi: 10.1016/j.ijpharm.2007.03.006.

Maione-Silva, L., de Castro, E.G., Nascimento, T.L., Cintra, E.R., Moreira, L.C., Cintra, B.A.S., Valadares, M.C., Lima, E.M., 2019. Ascorbic acid encapsulated into negatively charged liposomes exhibits increased skin permeation, retention and enhances collagen synthesis by fibroblasts. *Sci. Rep.* 9(1), 522.

Manca, M.L., Matricardi, P., Cencetti, C., Peris, J.E., Melis, V., Carbone, C., Escribano, E., Zaru, M., Fadda, A.M., Manconi, M., 2016. Combination of argan oil and phospholipids for the development of an effective liposome-like formulation able to improve skin hydration and allantoin dermal delivery. *Int. J. Pharm.* 505 (1–2), 204–211.

Manconi, M. *et al.*, 2018. Nanodesign of new self-assembling core-shell gellan-transfersomes loading baicalin and in vivo evaluation of repair response in skin. *Nanomed. Nanotechnol. Biol. Med.* 14(2), pp. 569–579. doi: 10.1016/j.nano.201 7.12.001.

Manosroi, A., Kongkaneramit, L., Manosroi, J., 2004. Stability and transdermal absorption of topical amphotericin B liposome formulations. *Int. J. Pharm.* 270, 279–286.

Masini, V., Bonte, F., Meybeck, A., Wepierre, J., 1993. Cutaneous bioavailability in hairless rats of tretinoin liposomes or gel. *J. Pharm. Sci.* 82, 17–21.

Mezei, M., Gulasekharam, V., 1980. Liposomes – a selective drug delivery system for topical route of administration. Lotion dosage form. *Life Sci.* 26, 1473–1477.

Mishra, D., Mishra, P.K., Dabadghao, S., Dubey, V., Nahar, M., Jain, N.K., 2010. Comparative evaluation of hepatitis B surface antigen-loaded elastic liposomes and ethosomes for human dendritic cell uptake and immune response. *Nanomedicine.* 6(1), 110–118.

Monti, D., Chetoni, P., Burgalassi, S., Tognetti, F., Najarro, M., Boldrini, E., Saettone, M.F., 2004. Liposome-encapsulated triamcinolone acetonide: in vitro/in vivo evaluation of the influence of formulation on release of triamcinolone acetonide. European Conference on Drug Delivery and Pharmaceutical Technology, Sevilla, Spain.

Montenegro, L., Panico, A.M., Ventimiglia, A., Bonina, F.P., 1996. In vitro retinoic acid release and skin permeation from different liposome formulations. *Int. J. Pharm.* 133, 89–96.

Moolakkadath, T., Aqil, M., Ahad, A., Imam, S.S., Praveen, A., Sultana, Y., Mujeeb, M., Iqbal, Z., 2019 Apr 5. Fisetin loaded binary ethosomes for management of skin cancer by dermal application on UV exposed mice. *Int. J. Pharm.* 560, 78–91. doi: 10.1016/j.ijpharm.2019.01.067.

Mostafa, M., Alaaeldin, E., Aly, U.F., Sarhan, H.A., 2018. Optimization and characterization of thymoquinone-loaded liposomes with enhanced topical antiinflammatory activity. *AAPS PharmSciTech.* 19(8), 3490–3500.

Mura, S., Pirot, F., Manconi, M., Falson F., Fadda A.M., 2007. Liposomes and niosomes as potential carriers for dermal delivery of minoxidil. *J. Drug Target.* 15(2), 101–108.

Nagle, A., Goyal, A.K., Kesarla, R., Murthy, R.R., 2011. Efficacy study of vesicular gel containing methotrexate and menthol combination on parakeratotic rat skin model. *J. Liposome Res.* 21(2), 134–140.

Natsheh, H., Vettorato, E., Touitou, E., 2019. Ethosomes for dermal administration of natural active molecules. *Curr. Pharm. Des.* 25(21), 2338–2348.

New, R.R.C., 1990. *Liposomes: A Practical Approach.* Oxford University Press, Oxford, New York, pp. 1–32.

Ogiso, T., Yamaguchi, T., Iwaki, M., Tanino, T., Miyake, Y., 2001. Effect of positively and negatively charged liposomes on skin permeation of drugs. *J. Drug Target.* 9, 49–59.

Oh, E.K., Jin S.E., Kim J.K., Park J.S., Park Y., Kim C.K., 2011. Retained topical delivery of 5-aminolevulinic acid using cationic ultradeformable liposomes for photodynamic therapy. *Eur. J. Pharm. Sci.* 44 (1–2): 149–157.

Omar, M.M., Hasan, O.A., El Sisi, A.M., 2019. Preparation and optimization of lidocaine transferosomal gel containing permeation enhancers: a promising approach for enhancement of skin permeation. *Int. J. Nanomed.* 14, 1551–1562.

Parnham, M., 1992. Liposome Phospholipids: Toxicological and Environmental Advantages. In: Braun-Falco, O., Korting, H.C., Maibach, H.I. (Eds.), *Liposome Dermatics.* Springer-Verlag, Berlin, pp. 57–65.

Patil, Y.P., Jadhav, S., 2014. Novel methods for liposome preparation. *Chem. Phys. Lipids.* 177, 8–18.

Patzelt, A., Lademann, J., 2015. The Increasing Importance of the Hair Follicle Route in Dermal and Transdermal Drug Delivery. In: Dragicevic N., Maibach H. (eds) *Percutaneous Penetration Enhancers Chemical Methods in Penetration Enhancement.* Springer, Berlin, Heidelberg.

Perez-Cullell, N., Coderch, L., de la Maza, A., Parra, J.L., Estelrich, J., 2000. Influence of the fluidity of liposome compositions on percutaneous absorption. *Drug Deliv.* 7, 7–13.

Planas, M.E., Gonzalez, P., Rodriguez, L., Sanchez, S., Cevc, G., 1992. Noninvasive percutaneous induction of topical analgesia by a new type of drug carrier, and prolongation of local pain insensitivity by anesthetic liposomes. *Anesth. Analg.* 75, 615–621.

Priyanka, K., Singh, S., 2014. A review on skin targeted delivery of bioactives as ultradeformable vesicles: overcoming the penetration problem. *Curr. Drug Targets* 15(2), 184–198.

Puglia, C., Esposito, E., Menegatti, E., Nastruzzi, C., Rizza, L., Cortesi, R., Bonina, F.,

2005. Effect of charge and lipid concentration on in-vivo percutaneous absorption of methyl nicotinate from liposomal vesicles. *J. Pharm. Pharmacol.* 57, 1169–1176.

Puglia, C., Bonina, F., Rizza, L., Cortesi, R., Merlotti, E., Drechsler, M., Mariani, P., Contado, C., Ravani, L., Esposito, E., 2010. Evaluation of percutaneous absorption of naproxen from different liposomal formulations. *J. Pharm Sci.* 99, 2819–2829.

Rao, Y., Zheng, F., Zhang, X., Gao, J., Liang, W., 2008. In vitro percutaneous permeation and skin accumulation of finasteride using vesicular ethosomal carriers. *AAPS PharmSciTech.* 9(3), 860–865. doi: 10.1208/s12249-008-9124-y.

Rattanapak, T., Young, K., Rades, T., Hook, S., 2012. Comparative study of liposomes, transfersomes, ethosomes and cubosomes for transcutaneous immunisation: characterisation and in vitro skin penetration. *J. Pharm. Pharmacol.* 64(11), 1560–1569. doi: 10.1111/j.2042-7158.2012.01535.x.

Raza, K., Singh, B., Lohan, S., Sharma, G., Negi, P., Yachha, Y., Katare, O.P., 2013. Nanolipoidal carriers of tretinoin with enhanced percutaneous absorption, photostability, biocompatibility and anti-psoriatic activity. *Int. J. Pharm.* 456, 65–72.

Riaz, M., Weiner, N., Martin, F., 1989. Liposomes. In: Lieberman, H.A., Rieger, M.M., Banker, G.S. (eds) *Pharmaceutical Dosage Forms: Disperse Sustems*, Vol. 2. Marcel Dekker, New York, Basel, pp. 567–603.

Rosoft, M., 1988. Specialized Pharmaceutical Emulsions. In: Liebermann, H.A., Rieger, M.M. (eds) *Pharmaceutical Dosage Forms: Disperse Systems*, Vol. 1. Marcel Dekker, New York-Basel, pp. 245–283.

Rukavina, Z., Šegvić Klarić, M., Filipović-Grčić, J., Lovrić, J., Vanić, Z., 2018. Azithromycin-loaded liposomes for enhanced topical treatment of methicillin-resistant Staphyloccocus aureus (MRSA) infections. *Int. J. Pharm.* 553(1-2), 109–119.

Sala, M., Diab, R., Elaissari, A., Fessi, H., 2018. Lipid nanocarriers as skin drug delivery systems: properties, mechanisms of skin interactions and medical applications. *Int. J. Pharm.* 535(1–2), 1–17.

Schaller, M., Korting, H.C., 1996. Interaction of liposomes with human skin: the role of the stratum corneum. *Adv. Drug Deliv. Rev.* 18, 303–309.

Schätzlein, A., Cevc, G., 1998. Non-uniform cellular packing of the stratum corneum and permeability barrier function of intant skin: a high-resolution confocal laser scanning microscopy study using highly deformable vesicles (Transfersomes). *Br. J. Dermatol.* 138, 583–592.

Schreier, H., Bouwstra, J., 1994. Liposomes and niosomes as topical drug carriers: dermal and transdermal drug delivery. *J. Control. Release* 30, 1–15.

Sessa, G., Weissmann, G.J., 1968. Phospholipid spherules (liposomes) as a model for biological membranes. *Lipid Res.* 9, 310–318.

Seth, A.K., Misra A., Umrigar D., 2004. Topical liposomal gel of idoxuridine for the treatment of herpes simplex: pharmaceutical and clinical implications. *Pharm. Dev. Technol.* 9(3), 277–289.

Sguizzato, M., Mariani, P., Spinozzi, F., Benedusi, M., Cervellati, F., Cortesi, R., Drechsler, M., Prieux, R., Valacchi, G., Esposito, E., 2020. Ethosomes for

Coenzyme Q10 Cutaneous Administration: From Design to 3D Skin Tissue Evaluation. *Antioxidants* 9(6), 485. doi: 10.3390/antiox9060485.

Shabana, S., Sailaja, A.K., 2015. Formulation and evaluation of diclofenac sodium transferosomes using different surfactants by thin film hydration method. *Der. Pharm. Lett.* 7, 43–53.

Shabana, S., Sailaja, A.K., 2015. Formulation and evaluation of diclofenac sodium transferosomes using different surfactants by thin film hydration method. *Der. Pharm. Lett.* 7, 43–53.

Shanmugam, S., Song, C.K., Nagayya-Sriraman, S., Baskaran, R., Yong, C.S., Choi, H.G., Kim, D.D., Woo, J.S., Yoo, B.K., 2009. Physicochemical characterization and skin permeation of liposome formulations containing clindamycin phosphate. *Arch. Pharm. Res.* 32, 1067–1075.

Sharma, A., Sharma, U.S., 1997. Liposomes in drug delivery: progress and limitations. *Int. J. Pharm.* 154, 123–140.

Shumilov, M., Touitou, E., 2010 Mar 15. Buspirone transdermal administration for menopausal syndromes, in vitro and in animal model studies. *Int. J. Pharm.* 387(1-2), 26–33. doi: 10.1016/j.ijpharm.2009.11.029.

Shumilov, M., Bercovich, R., Duchi, S., Ainbinder, D., Touitou, E., 2010 Oct. Ibuprofen transdermal ethosomal gel: characterization and efficiency in animal models. *J. Biomed. Nanotechnol.* 6(5), 569–576. doi: 10.1166/jbn.2010.1153.

Šiler-Marinkovic, S., 2016. Liposomes as drug delivery systems in dermal and transdermal drug delivery. In: Dragicevic, N., Maibach, H. (eds) *Percutaneous Penetration Enhancers Chemical Methods in Penetration Enhancement: Nanocarriers.* Springer, Berlin Heidelberg New York Dordrecht London, pp. 15–38.

Singh, H.P., Tiwary, A.K., Jain, S., 2010 Mar. Preparation and in vitro, in vivo characterization of elastic liposomes encapsulating cyclodextrin-colchicine complexes for topical delivery of colchicine. *Yakugaku Zasshi.* 130(3), 397–407. doi: 10.1248/yakushi.130.397. PMID: 20190524.

Sinico, C., Fadda, A.M., 2009. Vesicular carriers for dermal drug delivery. *Expert Opin. Drug Deliv.* 6, 813–825.

Škalko, N., Cajkovac, M., Jalsenjak, I., 1992. Liposomes with clindamycin hydrochloride in therapy of acne vulgaris. *Int. J. Pharm.* 85, 97–101.

Song, Y.K., Kim, C.K., 2006. Topical delivery of low-molecular-weight heparin with surface-charged flexible liposomes. *Biomaterials* 27, 271–280.

Tabbakhian, M., Tavakoli, N., Jaafari, M.R., Daneshamouz, S., 2006. Enhancement of follicular delivery of finasteride by liposomes and niosomes. 1. In vitro permeation and in vivo deposition studies using hamster flank and ear models. *Int. J. Pharm.* 323, 1–10

Thoma, K., Jocham, U.E., 1992. Liposome Dermatics: Assessment of Long-Term Stability. In: Braun-Falco, O., Korting, H.C., Maibach, H.I. (eds) *Liposome Dermatics.* Springer-Verlag, Berlin, pp. 150–166.

Touitou, E., Junginger, H.E., Weiner, N.D., Nagai, T., Mezei, M., 1994b. Liposomes as carriers for topical and transdermal delivery. *J. Pharm. Sci.* 83, 1189–1203.

Touitou, E., Levi-Schaffer, F., Dayan, N., Alhaique, F., Riccieri, F., 1994a.

Modulation of caffeine skin delivery by carrier design: liposomes versus permeation enhancers. *Int. J. Pharm.* 103, 131–136.

Touitou, E., Dayan, N., Bergelson, L., Godin, B., Eliaz, M., 2000. Ethosomes – novel vesicular carriers: characterization and delivery properties. *J. Control. Release* 65, 403–418.

Touitou, E., Shaco-Ezra, N., Dayan, N., Jushynski, M., Rafaeloff, R., Azoury, R., 1992. Dyphylline liposomes for delivery to the skin. *J. Pharm. Sci.* 81, 131–134.

Van den Bergh, B.A.I., Salomons-De Vries, I., Bouwstra, J.A., 1998. Interactions between liposomes and human stratum corneum studied by freeze-substitution electron microscopy. *Int. J. Pharm.* 167, 57–67.

Van den Bergh, B.A.I., Bouwstra, J.A., Junginger, H.E., Wertz, P.W., 1999a. Elasticity of vesicles affects hairless mouse skin structure and permeability. *J. Control. Release* 62, 367–379.

Van den Bergh, B.A.I., Vroom, J., Gerritsen, H., Junginger, H.E., Bouwstra, J.A., 1999b. Interactions of elastic and rigid vesicles with human skin in vitro: electron microscopy and two-photon excitation microscopy. *Biochim. Biophys. Acta* 1461, 155–173.

Van Kuijk-Meuwissen, M.E.M.J., Junginger, H.E., Bouwstra, J.A., 1998a. Interactions between liposomes and human skin in vitro, confocal laser scanning microscopy study. *Biochim. Biophys. Acta* 1371, 31–39.

Van Kuijk-Meuwissen, M.E.M.J., Mougin, L., Junginger, H.E., Bouwstra, J.A., 1998b. Application of vesicles to rat skin in vivo: a confocal laser scanning microscopy study. *J. Control. Release* 56, 189–196.

Verma, D.D., Verma, S., Blume, G., Fahr, A., 2003b. Liposomes increase skin penetration of entrapped and non-entrapped hidrophilic substances into human skin: a skin penetration and confocal laser scanning microscopy study. *Eur. J. Pharm. Biopharm.* 55, 271–277.

Verma, D.D., Verma, S., Blume, G., Fahr, A., 2003a. Particle size of liposomes influences dermal delivery of substances into skin. *Int. J. Pharm.* 258, 141–151.

Verma, D.D., Verma, S., McElwee, K.J., Freyschmidt-Paul, P., Hoffman, R., Fahr, A., 2004. Treatment of alopecia areata in the DEBR model using cyclosporin A lipid vesicles. *Eur. J. Dermatol.* 14, 332–338.

Walunj, M., Doppalapudi, S., Bulbake, U., Khan, W., 2020. Preparation, characterization, and *in vivo* evaluation of cyclosporine cationic liposomes for the treatment of psoriasis. *J. Liposome Res.* 30(1), 68–79.

Wang, W., Lu, K.J., Yu, C.H., Huang, Q.L., Du, Y.Z., 2019. Nano-drug delivery systems in wound treatment and skin regeneration. *J. Nanobiotechnol.* 17(1), 82.

Xu, H.L., Chen, P.P., ZhuGe, D.L., Zhu, Q.Y., Jin, B.H., Shen, B.X., Xiao, J., Zhao, Y.Z., 2017. Liposomes with silk fbroin hydrogel core to stabilize bFGF and promote the wound healing of mice with deep second-degree scald. *Adv. Healthc Mater.* 6

Yeung, C.K., Shek, S.Y., Yu, C.S., Kono, T., Chan, H.H., 2011. Liposome-encapsulated 0.5% 5-aminolevulinic acid with intense pulsed light for the treatment of inflammatory facial acne: a pilot study. *Dermatol. Surg.* 37(4), 450–459.

Yokomizo, Y., Sagitani, H., 1996a. Effects of phospholipids on the percutaneous penetration of indomethacin through the dorsal skin of guinea pigs in vitro. *J. Control. Release* 38, 267–274.

Yokomizo, Y., Sagitani, H., 1996b. Effects of phospholipids on the in vitro percutaneous penetration of prednisolone and analysis of mechanism by using attenuated total reflectance-Fourier transform infrared spectroscopy. *J. Pharm. Sci.* 85, 1220–1226.

Yu, H.Y., Liao, H.M., 1996. Triamcinolone permeation from different liposome formulations through rat skin in vitro. *Int. J. Pharm.* 127, 1–7.

Zellmer, S., Pfeil, W., Lasch, J., 1995. Interaction of phosphatidylcholine liposomes with the human stratum corneum. *Biochim. Biophys. Acta* 1237, 176–182.

Zhai, Y., Zhai, G., 2014. Advances in lipid-based colloid systems as drug carrier for topic delivery. *J. Control Release.* 193, 90–99.

Zhang, J.P., Wei, Y.H., Zhou, Y., Li, Y.Q., Wu, X.A., 2012. Ethosomes, binary ethosomes and transfersomes of terbinafine hydrochloride: a comparative study. *Arch. Pharm. Res.* 35(1), 109–117. doi: 10.1007/s12272-012-0112-0.

Zhang, Y., Ng, W., Hu J., Mussa, S.S., Ge, Y., Xu, H., 2018. Formulation and in vitro stability evaluation of ethosomal carbomer hydrogel for transdermal vaccine delivery. *Colloids Surf. B Biointerfaces.* 163, 184–191. doi: 10.1016/j.colsurfb. 2017.12.031.

Zhou, Y., Wei, Y.H., Zhang, G.Q., Wu, X.A., 2010 Apr. Synergistic penetration of ethosomes and lipophilic prodrug on the transdermal delivery of acyclovir. *Arch. Pharm. Res.* 33(4), 567–574. doi: 10.1007/s12272-010-0411-2.

Zou, L., Ding, W., Zhang, Y., Cheng, S., Li F., Ruan, R., Wei, P., Qiu, B., 2018. Peptide-modified vemurafenib-loaded liposomes for targeted inhibition of melanoma via the skin. *Biomaterials* 182, 1–12.

Invasomes for Dermal and Transdermal Drug Delivery

3

3.1 DEVELOPMENT OF INVASOMES

Conventional liposomes are used only for dermal drug delivery due to their inefficient transdermal drug delivery, thus, there was a need to develop a new generation of lipid-based vesicles. Different approaches were used to obtain novel vesicles with higher penetration enhancing ability. At the end, vesicles were obtained, which contain besides phospholipids in their bilayers, small amounts of edge activators, such as surfactants (e.g. polysorbate 80, polysorbate 20, etc.), ethanol, terpenes, etc. to enhance their membrane fluidity and deformability/elasticity, and hence their penetration enhancing ability. Because of their deformable bilayers, these vesicles were named *elastic, deformable* or *flexible vesicles*. These elastic liposomes, termed transfersomes – containing different surfactants (Cevc and Chopra, 2016; Ahmed, 2015; Khan et al., 2015; Al Shuwaili et al., 2016), ethosomes – containing high ethanol amounts (Ainbinder et al., 2010; Zhai et al., 2015; Abdulbaqi et al., 2016; Ainbinder et al., 2016; Garg et al., 2016), transethosomes – containing surfactants and ethanol (Ascenso et al., 2015), invasomes – containing terpenes and ethanol (Dragicevic-Curic et al., 2008; Dragicevic et al., 2016; Dragicevic-Curic et al., 2010; Dragicevic-Curic et al., 2009), are being investigated both for dermal and transdermal drug delivery. These vesicles have been studied as drug carriers for a range of small molecules, peptides, proteins and vaccines, both *in vitro* and *in vivo* (Benson, 2017). For a comprehensive review of different vesicles, the reader should refer to reference (Dragicevic and Maibach, 2016), while here invasomes will be discussed.

The novel type of nanocarriers termed by the inventors "invasomes" were developed in 2000s by the group of Prof. Alfred Fahr (Verma, 2002). The first used invasomes represented phospholipid vesicles, composed of 10% w/w unsaturated soya phosphatydilcholine (PC), 3.3% w/v ethanol, 0.5 or 1% w/v of a terpene mixture (cineole:citral:d-limonene = 0.45:0.45:0.10 v/v, penetration enhancer [PE]), named also the "standard terpene mixture", and phosphate buffer saline (PBS) up to 100% w/v. Besides the bilayer forming phospholipid PC, invasomes usually contain also a small amount of lysophosphatidylcholine as an edge activator to impart deformability to the vesicles. The later developed invasomes contained besides phospholipids and ethanol, not only the standard terpene mixture, but also other terpene mixtures, as well as different single terpenes (Dragicevic-Curic et al., 2009). Thus, newly developed invasomes may contain different phospholipids, as well as different terpenes (Figure 3.1).

The inventors used unsaturated phospholipids due to their low main transition temperature (T_m), which leads to the formation of liposomes with phospholipid membranes being in a liquid crystalline thermodynamic state. This was important due to the findings that liquid-state vesicles have proven to be superior to gel-state vesicles (Van Kuijk-Meuwissen et al., 1998; El Maghraby et al., 1999; El Maghraby et al., 2001). As this was not sufficient to obtain vesicles being highly efficient in enhancing skin penetration of drugs, the phospholipid membranes were further modified, with the aim to obtain deformable/elastic vesicles. Elastic vesicles have shown to be superior to conventional gel-state and even liquid-state vesicles in terms of interactions with human skin (Van Den Bergh et al., 1999) and enhanced drug penetration (El Maghraby et al., 1999). Thus, the authors added penetration enhancers, i.e.

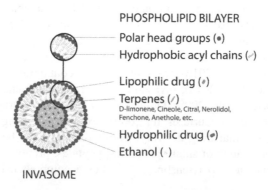

PHOSPHOLIPID BILAYER
- Polar head groups (●)
- Hydrophobic acyl chains (⌀)
- Lipophilic drug (●)
- Terpenes (∕)
  D-limonene, Cineole, Citral, Nerolidol, Fenchone, Anethole, etc.
- Hydrophilic drug (●)
- Ethanol ( )

INVASOME

FIGURE 3.1   Schematic presentation of structure and composition of invasomes.

terpenes and ethanol into the vesicles to enhance their fluidity and impart deformability to these carriers. Terpenes have been generally used as efficient penetration enhancers, as they increase the fluidity of *stratum corneum* (SC) lipid bilayers, and, thus, the penetration of drugs into/through the skin (Cornwell et al., 1994). It was supposed that terpenes would also increase the fluidity of vesicles' bilayers, i.e. their deformability, which was later confirmed by differential scanning calorimetry (DSC) (Dragicevic-Curic et al., 2011). The inventors added also ethanol in a small amount to liposomes, despite the assumption that ethanol is detrimental to liposomes, and is therefore usually removed from ethanolic solutions of phospholipids during the preparation of liposomes. Ethanol was added, as it was believed that it would fluidize the vesicles' bilayers in the same manner as it fluidizes the SC lipid bilayers, which was confirmed by Touitou et al. (2000) who developed ethosomes. Ethosomes represent vesicles containing besides phospholipids and water also high amounts of ethanol (>30%), being physically stable and able to deliver drugs to the deep skin layers and/or the systemic circulation (Godin and Touitou, 2003; Ainbinder and Touitou, 2005). In conclusion, the inventors of invasomes chose this interesting composition for their vesicles as they assumed that these potent penetration enhancers, ethanol and terpenes, would act synergistically on the fluidity and deformability of the vesicles' bilayers, as well as on disturbing the SC lipid bilayers. Further, they assumed that these chemical penetration enhancers could act synergistically with liposomes in enhancing the drug penetration into/through the skin.

3.2 TERPENES AS PENETRATION ENHANCERS ENCLOSED IN INVASOMES

Terpenes and essential oils have been extensively investigated for the penetration enhancement of different drugs due to their high penetration enhancing potential and low toxicity (Williams and Barry, 2004; Sapra et al., 2008). Terpenes are volatile substances derived from plant essential oils. They are reported to have good toxicological profiles, i.e. low cutaneous irritancy in the concentration range of 1–5% compared to synthetic penetration enhancers, such as Azone® (Yi et al., 2016; Xie et al., 2016; Lan et al., 2014). Their interaction with the SC lipids has been reported to be reversible (Okabe et al., 1990; Obata et al., 1991). The chemical structure of terpenes' molecules is

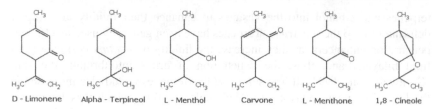

D - Limonene   Alpha - Terpineol   L - Menthol   Carvone   L - Menthone   1,8 - Cineole

FIGURE 3.2 Chemical structure of some terpenes.

based on repeated isoprene units (C_5H_8) (with exception of lavandulol), and hence they may be classified depending on the number of isoprene units into: monoterpenes (two isoprene units), sesquiterpenes (three isoprene units) or diterpenes (four isoprene units). Terpenes may be subdivided as acyclic, monocyclic, bicyclic, etc. In addition, terpenes are made up of various chemical classes such as hydrocarbons, alcohols, oxides and ketones (Williams and Barry, 2004). Chemical structures of some terpenes used as penetration enhancers are represented in Figure 3.2.

Terpenes have been used alone or in combination with ethanol or propylene glycol, to enhance the skin permeation of both lipophilic drugs, such as indomethacin (Levison et al., 1994), ketoprofen (Rhee et al., 2001), ibuprofen (Brain et al., 2005), estradiol (Monti et al., 2002), tamoxifen (El-Kattan et al., 2001), haloperidol (Vaddi et al., 2002; Vaddi et al., 2002), zidovudine (Narishetty and Panchagnula, 2004), hydrocortisone (El-Kattan et al., 2000), bulfalin (Yang et al., 2013) and hydrophilic drugs, including lidocaine hydrochloride (Sammeta et al., 2011), propranolol hydrochloride (Zhou et al., 2015; Cui et al., 2011) bupranolol (Babu and Pandit, 2005), 5-fluorouracil (Yi et al., 2016), nicardipine hydrochloride (Krishnaiah et al., 2003), and others.

The most extensively studied terpenes are D-limonene, 1.8-cineole and L-menthol, which have been used for penetration enhancement of both hydrophilic and lipophilic drugs (Aqil et al., 2007; Chen et al., 2016). However, other monoterpenes, such as anethol, carvacrol, carvone (Krishnaiah et al., 2003, 2004; Tas et al, 2007; Songkro et al., 2009), eucalyptol, alpha-pinene oxide, geraniol (Moghimi et al., 1997), linalool (Vaddi et al., 2002), etc. have been also investigated as penetration enhancers. In addition to small monoterpenes, larger terpene molecules (sesquiterpenes) have also been evaluated as penetration enhancers, such as nerolidol (Zhou et al., 2015) and farnesol (Nokhodchi et al., 2007). For more details on the use of terpenes refer to reference (Chen et al., 2016).

3.2.1 Structure-Activity Relationship of Terpenes

Williams and Barry (1991a,b) evaluated different monoterpenes as enhancers for 5-fluorouracil and confirmed a structure-activity relationship. Their data revealed that hydrocarbon terpenes were less potent enhancers for the hydrophilic drug 5-fluorouracil than the oxygen-containing terpenes (alcohols, ketones, oxides), which showed a moderate accelerant activity. Alcohols were generally less effective than ketones, while oxide terpenes induced the highest penetration enhancement (cyclic ethers being more potent than epoxides). Hence, the pre-treatment of human epidermal membranes with 1,8-cineole provided a nearly 100-fold increase in the permeability coefficient of 5-fluorouracil. This structure-activity relationship seemed to be drug specific, since results obtained with the lipophilic drug estradiol (Williams and Barry, 1991b) showed that, unlike for 5-flourouracil, where alcohol and ketone terpenes showed moderate enhancement activities, these same agents had no accelerent activity towards the lipophilic drug (they even retarded its permeation). The cyclic ethers, being extremely potent for 5-fluorouracil, induced only a moderate permeation enhancement of estradiol. In addition, hydrocarbon terpenes (such as D-limonene), being least effective for 5-fluorouracil, were the most effective enhancers for estradiol. These results were in accordance with results obtained for another lipophilic molecule, indomethacin, while hydrocarbon terpenes (especially limonene) were as effective as Azone® in promoting drug flux, and oxygen containing terpenes (carvone, 1,8-cineole) were ineffective (Okabe et al., 1989). It has been shown that among terpenes, hydrophilic terpenes (alcohols, ketones and oxide terpenes, like fenchone and thymol) are more effective in enhancing the permeation of hydrophilic drugs (propranolol), whereas, hydrocarbon lipophilic terpenes (like limonene and cymene) are most effective towards lipophilic drugs (diazepam) (Hori et al., 1991; Moghimi et al., 1997). In addition, anethole, a hydrophobic terpene, enhanced significantly the absorption of the highly lipophilic etodolac, while the hydrophilic terpenes, menthol and carvacrol, did not enhance the absorption of etodolac (Tas et al., 2007). Anethole with highest (log P) among different terpenes (log P = 3.39) provided the highest skin penetration of lipophilic valsartan (log P = 4.5), while eugenol (log P = 2.30) was the least effective penetration enhancer (Ahad et al., 2016). Hence, high lipophilicity of terpenes is important for enhancing the permeation of lipophilic drugs (Ghafourian et al., 2004). However, amphiphilic terpenes (such as nerolidol) possess a high penetration enhancing ability for most drugs due to their amphiphilic structure enabling the disruption of the highly organized lipid packing in the SC (Zhou et al., 2015; Erdal et al., 2014).

In a study with twelve sesquiterpene compounds, enhancers with polar functional groups were generally more potent than pure hydrocarbons in increasing the skin penetration of the hydrophilic drug 5-fluorouracil (Cornwell and Barry, 1994). Furthermore, enhancers with the least branched structures were the most active. The highest effect was observed following pretreatment with nerolidol, which increased pseudo-steady-state flux of 5-fluorouracil over 20-fold. In addition, molecular modeling suggested that sesquiterpenes with structures suitable for alignment within lipid lamellae were the most potent enhancers (Williams and Barry, 2004).

In addition, smaller terpenes tend to be more active penetration enhancers than the larger sesquiterpenes (Williams and Barry, 2004). It has also been observed that the (−) enantiomer of a terpene is a more effective penetration enhancer than the corresponding (±) racemate or the (+) isomer (Monti et al., 1995). Furthermore, the boiling point of a terpene is inversely related to its skin permeation enhancing capacity (Narishetty and Panchagnula, 2004). This can be attributed to the fact that terpenes with a low boiling point have relatively weaker intermolecular cohesive forces, and the oxygen of their functional group is mostly free, thus, available for hydrogen bonding between the functional groups of terpenes and the skin ceramides, thereby disrupting the packing of the SC lipids (Zhou et al., 2015). A similar inverse relationship exists between the energy of vaporization of a terpene and its penetration enhancing ability towards hydrophilic drugs (Ghafourian et al., 2004).

3.2.2 Lipophilicity of the Drug

More recent studies, investigating the impact of the *drug lipophilicity*, have shown a parabolic curve relationship between log P values of drugs and the enhancement ratio (ER) values of terpenes. The ER of limonene was in a parabolic curve relationship with the lipophilicity of drugs, indicating that limonene exhibits its highest penetration enhancing ability in the case of moderate lipophilic drugs (log P of 1.0) (Lan et al., 2014). As to borneol, a similar parabolic curve relationship between ER and log P values of drugs was seen, which proposed its optimum permeation enhancing ability for moderately hydrophilic drugs (log P of -0.5~0.5) (Yi et al., 2016). The same trend was observed for camphor, which showed that the most promising log P value of the drug was about zero to obtain the highest penetration enhancing effect of camphor (Xie et al., 2016). Thus, the terpenes represent potent penetration enhancers for hydrophilic and amphiphilic drugs rather than for hydrophobic drugs. These findings revealed the importance of both lipophilicity of drugs and terpenes.

3.2.3 Mechanism of Skin Penetration Enhancement by Terpenes

Terpenes increase the drug penetration into the skin by more than one mechanism of action. However, it is proposed that their interactions with SC intercellular lipids represent their key mechanism of action. Thus, terpenes may influence the SC lipids by acting at two sites, the lipophilic tails of the intercellular lipids and their polar head groups. They may also act by increasing the SC partitioning of the drug and/or by modifying the keratinized protein conformations since these are also the mechanisms of action of penetration enhancers (Williams and Barry, 2004).

In early studies it has been shown for hydrophilic drugs, such as 5-fluorouracil, that the primary effect of the terpenes' treatment is to increase drug diffusivity in the SC, i.e. to reduce the barrier properties of the skin (Cornwell et al., 1994; Williams and Barry, 1991b). The terpenes disrupt the lipid structure of the SC, thereby increasing the diffusion coefficient of the polar drug in the membrane, illustrated by the reduced lag time observed and diffusivity calculated from permeation studies. The terpenes do not increase the partitioning of the hydrophilic drug into the human SC, since 5-fluorouracil is less soluble in all terpenes than in water. The high log P values of terpenes imply that the penetration enhancers will not significantly modify corneocyte proteins (Cornwell et al., 1994; Williams and Barry, 1991b). For more lipophilic drugs, such as estradiol, terpenes increase drug diffusivity, but also increase drug partitioning into the SC (Williams and Barry, 1991b). The increase in partitioning is likely to be due to bulk solvent effects since estradiol is moderately soluble in many of the terpenes. The permeation of lipophilic drugs increases proportionally to their solubility in the enhancer (Williams and Barry, 1991b). Thus, as a positive correlation between terpene uptake (menthol, thymol, carvacrol, menthone, and cineole) into the SC intercellular lipids and β-estradiol partitioning enhancement was found, it has been proposed that terpene dissolved in the intercellular lipid domain can help to improve drug partitioning into the SC (Chantasart et al., 2009). Further, the interaction between the drug and terpenes via hydrogen bonding was proposed to contribute to the enhancement of the partition coefficient (Cui et al., 2011). However, as aforementioned, the SC partition of drugs is markedly influenced by the lipophilicity of the drug, as it has been shown that lipophilic camphor among drugs of different lipophilicities (log P from -0.48 to 3.8) enhanced at most the partition of lipophilic drugs into the SC (Xie et al., 2016).

Abd et al. investigated the influence of eucalyptol and oleic acid on the permeation of caffeine and naproxen (Abd et al., 2019). They suggested that increased drug diffusivity was the main driving force which increased the permeation flux of the hydrophilic molecule caffeine, rather than effects on SC solubility, while for the more lipophilic drug naproxen, increased SC solubility was responsible for the increased drug permeation flux.

The mechanism by which terpenes act on the SC lipids and increase drug diffusivity has been investigated by different techniques. DSC measurements have shown that terpenes reduce lipid phase transition temperatures (T_m), implying that they may increase SC permeability by disrupting the intercellular lipid bilayers (Cornwell et al., 1994; Williams and Barry, 1989). DSC studies with 1.8-cineole, D-limonene, menthone and nerolidol in propylene glycol/water systems, provided evidence that 1.8-cineole, menthone and nerolidol are lipid disruptive, whereas they provided no clear proof of a lipid disruptive effect of D-limonene (Yamane et al., 1995; Cornwell et al., 1996). D-Limonene produced a freezing point-depression effect on the SC lipids, suggesting little interaction with lipids at skin temperature in contrast to the high enhancement effect achieved by 1.8-cineole, menthone and nerolidol, and its small enhancement effect may involve phase separation of the oil in SC lipids (Yamane et al., 1995; Cornwell et al., 1996). However, small angle X-ray diffraction (SAXD) studies have indicated that D-limonene and 1,8-cineole disrupt SC bilayer lipids (i.e. induce reductions in bilayer periodicity), whereas nerolidol (a long chain sesquiterpene) reinforces the bilayers, possibly by orienting alongside the SC lipids (Cornwell et al., 1996). SAXD and wide angle X-ray diffraction (WAXD) measurements have confirmed that D-limonene caused a slight disruption of the organized lipid bilayers' structures (the hexagonal hydrocarbon-chain packing structure was much strongly disrupted than the orthorhombic one), an increase of the repeat distance of the long lamellar structure by incorporating D-limonene molecules, and formation of "pools" of D-limonene in the hydrophobic region of the intercellular lipid matrix in the SC (Hatta et al., 2010). Regarding L-menthol, SAXD and WAXD studies investigated its effect on the behavior of ceramide 2/cholesterol mixtures (used as a model for the intercellular lipids in the SC) and revealed that, it increased the repeat distance of the lamellar structure and inhibited the formation of hexagonal hydrocarbon chain packing. Moreover, DSC studies showed that it decreased the phase transition temperature of ceramide 2/cholesterol mixtures. Hence, L-menthol changed the lamellar structure and the intermolecular interaction between ceramide 2 and cholesterol. These effects of L-menthol are related to fluidization of lipid structures of ceramide 2/cholesterol mixtures and help promote the transdermal drug permeation (Watanabe et al., 2009).

Attenuated total reflection-Fourier transform infrared spectroscopy (ATR-FTIR) or FT-IR spectrometry are often used to clarify the mechanism of action of penetration enhancers as they investigate alterations of the skin barrier by obtaining the conformation information of the SC lipids and keratins. The shift of stretching peaks (C-H symmetric stretching absorbance frequency peak; C-H asymmetric stretching absorbance frequency peak; Amide I; Amide II) is usually detected following the administration of terpenes onto the SC, i.e. shift to a higher frequency of C-H stretching peaks indicates the perturbation of SC lipids. The stronger the perturbation, the higher the C-H stretching peak position. In addition, extraction of the lipids by terpenes results always in a decrease of peak area and peak height (Hoppel et al., 2014). Thus, ATR-FTIR revealed that administration of L-menthol caused disorder of the intercellular lipids in the SC similar to that of heat application (Obata et al., 2010), which was already proposed by other authors (Watanabe et al., 2009). DSC and ATR-FTIR studies with 1,8-cineole and L-menthol revealed that both terpenes exerted effects on both lipid acyl tails and polar head groups, as demonstrated by a reduction in the main transition temperature (T_m) and in the nonhydrogen bonded amide I stretching frequency, respectively (Narishetty and Panchagnula, 2005). The results suggested, however, that at physiological temperature, terpenes mainly act at polar head groups and break the inter- and intralamellar hydrogen bonding network, leading to decreased integrity in the SC barrier. Terpenes also increased the hydration levels of the lipid system probably by forming new aqueous channels. These results indicated that 1.8-cineole and L-menthol enhanced transdermal permeation of zidovudine by transforming SC lipids from a highly ordered orthorhombic perpendicular subcellular packing to a less ordered hexagonal subcell packing. FTIR studies revealed the permeation enhancement of nicorandil by nerolidol and carvone due to partial lipid extraction (Krishnaiah et al., 2006), propranolol hydrochloride by menthone and D-limonene (combination with ethanol) due to lipid extraction, macroscopic barrier perturbations, and increased partitioning of the drug into the SC (Zhao and Singh, 1999), and tamoxifen by eugenol and D-limonene (combination with ethanol) due to lipid extraction and increased partitioning and by menthone only due to lipid extraction (Zhao and Singh, 1998). A similar FTIR study showed that the enhanced permeability of the SC to tamoxifen by menthone, eugenol, and limonene (combination with propylene glycol) was due to lipid extraction and macroscopic barrier perturbation. Moreover, the effective diffusion coefficient of tamoxifen through the epidermis was enhanced following treatment with either eugenol or limonene (Zhao and Singh, 1998). FTIR and DSC studies revealed that the diterpene forskolin enhanced skin permeation of valsartan by disruption and extraction of lipid bilayers of the SC (Rizwan et al., 2008).

Recent ATR-FTIR studies showed that menthol and menthone could only slightly interact with the lipophilic tails of skin lipids. However, menthol and menthone led to a significant decrease of peak areas of C-H stretching absorption peaks, confirming their ability to extract part of the SC lipids, thereby weakening the SC permeability barrier. In addition, as no significant difference in the peak positions/areas of two amide bonds was seen, it was concluded that these terpenes had a minor effect on the keratin in corneocytes (Lan et al., 2016). Menthone showed a higher capacity in disturbing and extracting lipids than menthol and Azone® (Wang et al., 2017). As to other terpenes 1,8-cineole, 1,4-cineole, rose oxide, safranal, and valencene, ATR-FTIR showed that they enhanced permeation of valsartan by directly extracting SC lipids, as height and area of stretching peaks decreased (Ahad et al., 2011), while that they did not fluidize the SC lipids (no shift of peaks to higher wave number was seen) (Ahad et al., 2011). In contrast, nerolidol fluidized mainly the SC lipids, while less extracting them (Erdal et al., 2014).

Regarding the effect of terpenes on the hydrogen bonds between ceramides, it also contributes to the penetration enhancing ability of terpenes. Namely, ceramides are tightly packed in the SC lipid bilayer by hydrogen bonding, which makes the SC lipid bilayer strong in order to maintain the permeability barrier of the SC. However, this tight network may be weakened by terpenes with a functional group that can donate or accept a hydrogen bond. It has been shown by using FTIR that, terpenes with weak self-association or which have the ability of donating or accepting H-bonds (like menthol, cineole, menthone) increase the permeation of a watersoluble, polar drug, imipramine hydrochloride, through the breaking of hydrogen bonds between ceramides' polar head groups (Jain et al., 2002). These findings were confirmed also in other studies (Narishetty and Panchagnula, 2005; Wang et al., 2017).

It has also been shown that, following enhancer treatment, liquid terpenes are incorporated in the SC in high quantities, and they are phase-separated within the SC from undisrupted lipid bilayers, i.e. they could exist within separate domains in the SC (Cornwell et al., 1994, 1996). According to Cornwell et al. (1996), a proportion of terpenes may form droplets in the intercellular lipid domains. In addition to this mechanism, a proportion may distribute into the corneocytes. Despite higher partitioning of terpenes into the lipid domains, their uptake into the protein domains may be significant due to the fact that intracellular protein domains make up 70–95% of the SC volume.

The permeation enhancement of mefenamic acid by 1,8-cineole was due to a "drag" or "pull" effect (Heard et al., 2006).

3.2.4 Synergistic Action of Terpenes With Co-Solvents

Terpenes, used together with propylene glycol show a higher enhancer efficacy, because of their synergistic effect (Chen et al., 2016). It was reported that the enhancer efficacies for carveol, carvone, pulegone, and 1,8-cineole rose approximately 4-fold when used with propylene glycol (Williams and Barry, 1989).

Terpenes' (1,8-cineole, menthone, (+)-limonene and nerolidol,) activity depended on the propylene glycol content in the vehicles and maximum fluxes of 5-fluorouracil were obtained from formulations containing terpenes in 80% propylene glycol systems (Yamane et al., 1995). The combination menthol/propylene glycol enhanced the permeation of propofol (Yamato et al., 2009) and imipramine hydrochloride (Shah et al., 2008). Further, the combination of menthone, menthol, or pulegone with propylene glycol significantly increased the penetration of drugs of different lipophilicities, by perturbing and extracting the SC lipids (Lan et al., 2016). Limonene also increased the penetration of drugs of different lipophilicities from a propylene glycol vehicle by the same proposed mechanism (Lan et al., 2014). DSC and SAXD investigations provided fragmented evidence that terpene/propylene glycol synergy may produce enhanced lipid bilayer disruption (Cornwell et al., 1996). It has been proposed that propylene glycol is promoting the passage of terpenes into SC where they exert their accelerant activity. Thus, propylene glycol acts also by increasing the partitioning of the enhancer into the SC (Williams and Barry, 1989).

As to terpenes combined with ethanol, 1,8-cineole and L-menthol applied at 5% w/v in 66.6% ethanol as a vehicle significantly enhanced the pseudo steady-state flux of zidovudine (Narishetty and Panchagnula, 2005). Menthone (1,2,3 and 5%) in combination with 50% ethanol (Zhao et al., 2001) and 5% w/v of other terpenes (carvone, 1.8-cineole, menthol, and thymol) in 50% ethanol (Gao and Singh, 1998) significantly enhanced the flux of tamoxifen compared to the control (50% ethanol). The combination of 3% w/w 1.8-cineole and 47% w/w ethanol enhanced the permeation of the thyrotropin-releasing hormone (TRH) *in vitro* through rat skin and induced systemic effects *in vivo* in rats. Further, 1.8-cineole has shown to be effective in enhancing the permeation rate of propranolol hydrochloride and valsartan from ethanol: isotonic PBS pH 7.4 vehicle (40:60) (Ahad et al., 2011). Camphor used in PG:water (70:30) vehicle has been shown to increase the skin permeation of drugs with different lipophilicity (log P from 3.80 to -0.95), such as indomethacin, lidocaine, antipyrine, acetyl salicylic acid, tegafur, and 5-fluorocuracil, by approximately 4-, 6- 10-, 18-, 16-, 12-fold compared to the control (Xie et al., 2016). It has been shown that ethanol had a synergistic effect on the activity of terpenes in enhancing the percutaneous permeation of ketoprofen from different gel formulations (El-Kattan et al., 2000).

3.3 ETHANOL

Ethanol has been used as a vehicle in the pharmaceutical and cosmetics industries for many years. Ethanol alone or in combination with other chemical penetration enhancers and physical methods has been reported to be an efficient skin penetration enhancer (Morimoto et al., 2002; Morimoto et al., 2000; Joo et al., 2008). It has shown to be effective in enhancing the flux of levonorgestrel, estradiol, hydrocortisone, and 5-fluorouracil through rat skin *in vitro* (Williams and Barry, 2004), hinokitiol through hairless mouse skin *in vitro* (Joo et al., 2008). It has been used in the concentration of 5–96%, and several reports suggested that the effect of ethanol on the SC is concentration-dependent. The diffusion of the salicylate ion across human epidermal membranes was enhanced up to ethanol: water ratio of 0.63, whereas higher levels of ethanol decreased its permeation (Kurihara-Bergstrom et al., 1990). Similar results have been reported for zidovudine (Thomas and Panchagnula, 2003). It has been reported that the permeation of lipophilic drugs was enhanced using ethanol at lower concentrations, i.e. ethanol at 65% v/v was able to increase the permeation of fluoxetine at the most, while ethanol at 40% provided the highest skin penetration of cyclosporine A, in the following order ethanol 40% > ethyl oleate > Transcutol® > isopropyl myristate > ethanol > Labrasol® > propylene glycol > Lauroglycol FCC® (Parikh and Ghosh, 2005; Liu et al., 2006). Ethanol leads to lipid and protein extraction from the SC when used at high concentrations, i.e. 75% v/v (Goates and Knutson, 1994). FTIR study has shown that lipid extraction increased with increasing alcohol chain length, while SC protein conformation was significantly altered in the presence of already short chain alcohols, further increasing with the increase of alcohol chain length. Ethanol may cause also dehydration of the SC (Megrab et al., 1995), when used as absolute. It is proposed that the dehydration of the biological membrane which occurs at higher ethanol concentrations, reduced drug permeation across the skin (Williams and Barry, 2004). It has been shown in human and porcine skin *ex vivo* that ethanol: PBS (1:1) was the best-suited solvent for delivering the spin probe deep into the skin compared to absolute ethanol and PBS (Dong et al., 2020).

Ethanol can exert its permeation enhancing activity through various mechanisms. It disrupts the SC lipid organization (i.e. fluidizes the SC lipids), making it permeable. Ethanol and other penetration enhancers, which act in this way, penetrate into the SC bilayers, where they rotate, vibrate and form microcavities, thereby increasing the free volume for drug diffusion (Barry, 2001). As a solvent, it can increase the solubility of the drug in the vehicle, although at steady-state the flux of a permeant from any saturated, non-enhancing, vehicle should be equivalent. However, for poorly soluble permeants that are prone to deplete within the donor during a steady-state permeation study, ethanol can increase permeant solubility in the donor phase (Pershing et al., 1990). In addition, ethanol permeates into the SC and alters the solubility properties of the tissue resulting in an improvement of drug partitioning into the membrane

(Megrab et al., 1995). Further, due to the evaporation of ethanol from the donor phase, an increase of the thermodynamic activity of the drug within the formulation occurs, i.e. the drug concentration increases beyond saturated solubility providing a supersaturated state with a greater driving force for permeation. This mechanism is known as the "push effect" (Kadir and Stempler, 1987), and it may be responsible for transdermal delivery of drugs from patches where ethanol is included. It has also been suggested that ethanol, for which rapid permeation across the skin has been reported, could "pull" or "drag" the permeant with it (Heard et al., 2006), although such a mechanism has been discounted for morphine hydrochloride permeation from ethanol and methanol containing formulations (Morimoto et al., 2002). Ethanol as a volatile solvent may also extract some of the lipid fraction from within the SC, when used at high concentration for prolonged times, which improves drug flux through skin (Williams and Barry, 2004). Thermogravimetric analysis (TGA) and FTIR spectroscopy revealed that the application of ethanol dehydrated skin. It was confirmed that ethanol decreased the bound water content due to extraction of the SC lipids. In addition, ethanol (and propylene glycol) increased the permeation of solute and TEWL by dehydration, and the partition was predominant for the permeation of solute through dehydrated skin (Shah et al., 2008). SAXD and WAXD measurements showed that when the hydrophilic penetration enhancer, ethanol, was applied to the SC, a slight disruption of the organized lipid structures occurred, and among them the orthorhombic hydrocarbon-chain packing structure was disrupted more strongly (Hatta et al., 2010). Further, the structure of the soft keratin in the corneocytes was partially disrupted, which indicated that ethanol molecule penetrated through the corneocytes. In addition, ethanol pools seem to be formed in the intercellular lipid matrix. These results indicate that ethanol yields transcellular routes through which hydrophilic molecules penetrate (Hatta et al., 2010).

As to the influence of ethanol on phospholipid liposomes, regarding its potential to fluidize the vesicles' bilayers, it has been shown that the addition of ethanol into DMPC liposomes led to a decrease of the transition temperatures of the phospholipid bilayers and the peak of the pre-transition was broadened (addition of 3.3% ethanol) or had disappeared completely (addition of 10% ethanol). The decreased pre-transition temperature of the DMPC vesicles upon addition of ethanol may point to molecular interactions between ethanol and the polar head groups of DMPC, resulting in increased mobility in the head group region of the phospholipid bilayer. The decreased main transition temperature indicated an increased molecular motion of the acyl chains and thus looser and more flexible bilayers (Dragicevic-Curic et al., 2011). Thus, ethanol increases the fluidity of vesicles (Ainbinder et al., 2016).

Ethanol as a penetration enhancer exhibits synergistic penetration enhancement with phospholipids as shown in the study with cyclosporine

A-loaded liposomes (Verma and Fahr, 2004). Thus, in the last decades, numerous studies have been devoted to the development of different ethanol-containing liposomes (ethosomes) encapsulating various drug substances (Ainbinder et al., 2016).

As to the influence of ethanol on vesicles' properties, ethanol decreases the vesicle size and drug entrapment efficiency upon increasing its concentration (see section 3.4). Further, an increase of ethanol amount in vesicles leads to the solubilization of vesicles. In addition, ethanol interpenetrates into the vesicles' bilayers and imparts a negative surface charge to vesicles (Dragicevic-Curic et al., 2010).

3.4 PREPARATION, PHYSICO-CHEMICAL PROPERTIES AND STABILITY OF INVASOMES

3.4.1 Preparation of Invasomes

Invasomes are most often prepared by the method of *mechanical dispersion*, as follows: the drug (lipophilic) and terpenes or mixtures of terpenes are dissolved in the ethanolic phospholipid solution, as mostly commercial mixtures of PC in ethanol are used (e.g. PC:ethanol = 75:25 w/w). The mixture is then vortexed for 5 min and sonicated for 5 min in order to obtain a clear solution. Afterwards phosphate buffer saline (PBS) pH 7.4 is added to 100% w/v to the solution for hydration of the vesicles under constant vortexing, which is continued for an additional 5 min. If a hydrophilic drug is encapsulated, it is dissolved in PBS. The last step is the extrusion of multilamellar vesicles through polycarbonate membranes of different pore sizes (400 nm, 200 nm, 100 nm, 50 nm), through each polycarbonate membrane 21 times. The formulations are extruded without removing ethanol in order to obtain vesicle dispersions containing 3.3% w/v ethanol (Dragicevic-Curic et al., 2008; Dragicevic-Curic et al., 2009; Verma et al., 2004).

Invasomes can also be prepared by the conventional film method. The lipophilic drug and phospholipids are dissolved in mixture of methanol:-chloroform (2:1, v/v). This mixture is dried to a thin film by slowly reducing the pressure from 500 to 1 mbar at 50 °C using the rotary evaporator. The film is kept under vacuum (1 mbar) for 2 h at room temperature and subsequently flushed with nitrogen. Then, the film is hydrated for 30 min at 50 °C with PBS (pH 7.4). After cooling to room temperature, ethanol and a single terpene or a terpene mixture are added in order to obtain invasomes. The obtained vesicles are vortexed, ultrasonicated and subsequently sized by 21 times extrusion through polycarbonate membranes of different pore sizes (400 nm, 200 nm, 100 nm, and 50 nm) (Dragicevic-Curic et al., 2011).

3.4.2 Characterization of Invasomes

The physico-chemical characterization of vesicles generally, i.e. determining their particle size, homogeneity (polydispersity index (PDI)), lamellarity, shape, zeta potential, encapsulation efficiency (EE%), drug content, pH value of dispersions, etc. is very important for their development, as some of these properties have an impact on the stability of vesicles, while some have on their ability to enhance the penetration of encapsulated drugs into/through the skin, and, hence, on their therapeutic effectiveness. Thus, the characterization of invasomes, especially for medical use is of crucial importance.

Regarding particle size of invasomes, it has been shown in temoporfin (mTHPC)-loaded invasomes that the addition of terpenes to liposomes containing 3.3% w/v ethanol had an impact on their physical properties, especially vesicle size. The increase of the amount of the standard terpene mixture increased the vesicle size of invasomes. However, despite the fact that terpenes increased the vesicle size, both types of mTHPC-invasomes, containing 0.5% w/v or 1% w/v terpene mixture, were of sufficiently small particle size, i.e. 93 nm and 124 nm, respectively (Dragicevic-Curic et al., 2008). An increase of particle size upon enhancing the amount of terpenes in invasomes was also observed in cyclosporine (CsA)-loaded invasomes (Verma, 2002), as well as in isradipine-loaded invasomes, as formulations bearing 0.1% β-citronellene showed smaller vesicles' particle size compared to formulations, containing 0.5% β-citronellene (Qadri et al., 2017). In the case of CsA-loaded invasomes with different terpene concentrations, they possessed particle size less than 100 nm till the concentration of PE ≤ 1%, however above this concentration the hand extruder was not able to produce CsA-loaded invasomes with vesicle size ≤100 nm (Verma, 2002). Ferulic-acid loaded invasomes with 1% standard terpene mixture possessed almost the same particle size (129 nm) as mTHPC-loaded invasomes with 1% w/v standard terpene mixture, and they were also negatively charged (Chen et al., 2010). As to the particle size of different invasomes with encapsulated hydrophilic dyes (such as carboxyfluorescein), it was also ranging between 95 nm (1% w/v cineole) and 132 nm (1.5% v/w standard terpene mixture) (Ntimenou et al., 2012). An increase of particle size of liposomes, when terpenes were added compared to liposomes without terpenes, was also seen for nimesulide-loaded invasomes. Further, nimesulide-loaded invasomes containing 1% citral, 1% limonene or

1% cineole possessed particle size of 194 nm, 216 nm and 255 nm, respectively, revealing also the influence of the type of terpene added on the particle size, wherein the negative surface charge of liposomes with ethanol (but without terpenes) did not vary much on the incorporation of the terpene and its increase in percentage (Badran et al., 2012). The incorporation of terpenes into ethosomes in order to obtain invasomes led to an increase in the vesicle size (and PDI values), showing a direct correlation between the terpene concentration and the vesicle size, which was in the range of 139.3 to 172.5 nm, being still low (Ammar et al., 2020). In addition, the particle size of agomelatine-loaded invasomes was significantly affected by the terpene type and concentration. Increasing the terpene concentration from 0.75% w/v to 1.5% w/v led to a significant increase in particle size of invasomes loaded with agomelatine (Tawfik et al., 2020). This could be referred to the ability of invasomes to accommodate more drug at a higher terpene concentration. An inverse correlation could be established between particle size and terpene's lipophilicity. Invasomes containing limonene possessed the lowest particle size compared to other invasomes. The authors attributed this to the greatest lipophilic property (log P = 4.83) of limonene among other terpenes, considering the concept of "like dissolves like", as the small particle size of invasomes containing limonene could be correlated to the matched lipophilic properties of the drug, PC, and limonene (Tawfik et al., 2020). Similar findings were reported by Saffari et al., who showed that limonene-based invasomes were smaller in size than cineole-based ones (Saffari et al., 2016). The type of added terpene influenced the vesicle size of avanafil-loaded invasomes, where D-limonene caused a significant reduction in the vesicle size compared to β-citronellol (Ahmed and Badr-Eldin, 2019). The authors explained this by the difference in the molecular weight and the lipophilicity of the terpenes used. Namely, invasomes containing β-citronellol (MW 156.27 g/mol) exhibited a larger vesicle size than those prepared using D-limonene (MW 136.24 g/mol). Further, β-citronellol (log P = 3.2) has lower lipophilicity than d-limonene (log P = 4.83), which could increase the repulsion force between the lipophilic components of vesicles and the terpene, thereby increasing the vesicular size of invasomes. Similar results were found by other authors (Saffari et al., 2016), who showed that liposomes of smaller vesicle size were obtained when D-limonene was used compared to the more hydrophilic terpene, cineole. Similarly, the smallest size for dapsone-loaded invasomes was obtained when using limonene compared to less lipophilic terpenes, such as cineole, citral and fenchone (El-Nabarawi et al., 2018).

However, in the case of some invasomes, terpenes did not affect the vesicle size, as seen in isotretinoin invasomes where the concentration of eugenol did not affect the vesicle size of invasomes (Dwivedi et al., 2017). Moreover, the particle size of finasteride-loaded invasomes (being in μm range) did not vary much with increasing the concentration of different terpenes (limonene, nerolidol, carvone) from 0.5 to 1.5%, while their entrapment efficiency showed an inverse relationship, i.e. it decreased as the terpene concentration increased. However, the authors attributed this to the different molecular weight of terpenes (limonene (MW 136.24 g/mol), carvone (MW 150.22 g/mol), and nerolidol (MW 222.37 g/mol)), wherein nerolidol of the largest molecular weight gave larger invasomes compared to limonene and carvone, having a smaller molecular weight (Ahmed and Rizq, 2018).

The particle size of invasomes was influenced by the phospholipid concentration since it increased with increasing phospholipid concentration, as shown for avanafil-loaded invasomes (Ahmed and Badr-Eldin, 2019), isotretinoin-loaded invasomes (Dwivedi et al., 2017), olmesartan-loaded invasomes (Kamran et al., 2016) and agomelatine-loaded invasomes (Tawfik et al., 2020). This was observed also for other types of vesicles, e.g. ethosomes loaded with an anti-psoriatic agent (Dubey et al., 2007). Tawfik et al. (2020) attributed the higher particle size of agomelatine-loaded invasomes comprising high lipid content, to the higher viscosities of the invasomal dispersions at the higher lipid concentration, which would lead to higher mass transfer resistances, lower sonication efficiencies, and, thus, larger particles, while Dwivedi et al. (2017) proposed that at a higher concentration of lecithin, the single hydrophobic chain with a polar head group of egg lecithin resulted in a highly positive curvature in membranes, which increased the invasomes' particle size. Regarding ethosomes (which were used to prepare invasomes), an indirect correlation between PC concentration and vesicle size was observed, where the increase of PC concentration, at constant ethanol concentration, decreased the vesicle size of ethosomes. The authors explained the decrease of vesicle size at high PC concentrations as a result of a reduction in the interfacial tension between the water and lipid phases due to high PC concentration, which also stabilizes the vesicles by providing steric barriers on their surfaces and thereby, protects them from aggregation (Ammar et al., 2020). In contrast to PC concentration, ethanol concentration at constant PC concentration did not show a significant effect on the vesicle size. The subsequent incorporation of terpenes into ethosomes led to an increase in the vesicle size (and PDI values), showing a direct correlation between the terpene concentration and the vesicle size, which was in the range of 139.3 to 172.5 nm. The goal in the development of vesicles is to obtain a small particle size of vesicles, in the nanometer range, since Verma et al. showed that the skin penetration of hydrophilic as well as lipophilic substances was inversely related to the size of liposomes (Verma et al., 2003). Thus, most developed invasomes were of sufficiently small particle size, possessing the prerequisite to efficiently interact with the SC and enhance the percutaneous drug penetration.

As to the homogeneity, invasome dispersions were of high homogeneity, since the PDI was mostly <0.2 (Dragicevic-Curic et al., 2008; Dragicevic-Curic et al., 2009; Verma, 2002; Chen et al., 2010; Ntimenou et al., 2012; Badran et al., 2012; Verma et al., 2003). Tawfik et al. (2020) found a direct correlation between the particle size and the PDI, and except for citral-based invasomes, all systems had PDI values <0.3.

The addition of terpenes had no effect on the lamellarity of invasomes as cryo-electron microscopy revealed that most vesicles were unilamellar and to a lesser extent also bilamellar, regardless if the terpenes were present in the vesicles' bilayer or not (Dragicevic-Curic et al., 2008; Dragicevic-Curic et al., 2009; Ntimenou et al., 2012; Badran et al., 2012; Verma et al., 2003). Azelaic acid-loaded and idebenone-loaded invasomes were mostly unilamellar showing a mixture of small unilamellar vesicles (SUVs) and large unilamellar vesicles (LUVs), although a few vesicles were oligolamellar (Shah et al., 2015). As to the shape of vesicles, in the case of mTHPC-loaded invasomes, the addition of terpenes had a strong influence (Dragicevic-Curic et al., 2008; Dragicevic-Curic et al., 2009). A detailed cryo-electron microscopic study revealed that besides spherical vesicles in mTHPC-loaded invasome dispersions, also deformed vesicles of different shapes were present, and an increase of the terpenes' amount resulted in their increased number (Figure 3.3). The deformed vesicles represented mostly unilamellar vesicles, however, with invaginations (Figure 3.3). The presence of invaginations was confirmed by

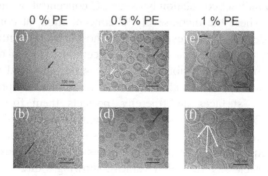

FIGURE 3.3 Visualization of mTHPC-liposomes containing 3.3% w/v ethanol and mTHPC-invasomes containing 0.5 and 1% w/v terpenes by cryo-electron microscopy.(a,b) mTHPC-liposomes with 3.3% w/v ethanol, (c, d) mTHPC-invasomes with 0.5% w/v terpenes, (e, f) mTHPC-invasomes with 1% w/v terpenes. Standard terpene mixture was used. Black short arrows represent unilamellar vesicles, black arrows of medium length represent bilamellar vesicles, while black long arrows represent oligolamellar vesicles. White arrows represent deformed vesicles (Dragicevic-Curic et al., 2008).

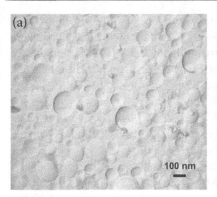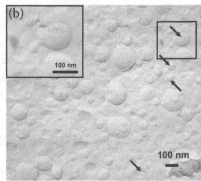

FIGURE 3.4 Visualization of mTHPC-invasomes with 1% w/v terpenes by freeze-fracture electron microscopy. (a) mTHPC-invasomes containing 1% w/v terpenes after preparation, (b) mTHPC-invasomes containing 1% w/v terpenes, 6 months after the preparation (stored at RT). Standard terpene mixture was used (Dragicevic-Curic et al., 2008).

freeze-fracture electron microscopy (Figure 3.4). This phenomenon was also seen in ferulic acid-loaded invasomes (Chen et al., 2010). It was assumed that the addition of terpenes, especially higher amounts, such as 1% w/v terpenes, to already liquid-state (fluid) liposomes with 3.3% w/v ethanol increased further their membrane deformability and fluidity, leading to the formation of deformed vesicles. The high membrane fluidity of mTHPC-loaded invasomes compared to mTHPC-loaded liposomes without terpenes was confirmed by DSC and electron spin resonance (ESR) measurements (Dragicevic-Curic et al., 2011).

Invasomes generally possess a negative surface charge, as shown by invasomes loaded with different drugs, which is attributed to the presence of ethanol imparting a negative surface charge to vesicles (Dragicevic-Curic et al., 2008; Tawfik et al., 2020; El-Nabarawi et al., 2018). In addition, the positively charged choline group of PC could be oriented to the inside, while the negatively charged phosphatidyl group of PC could be positioned to the outside of the bilayers, resulting in a high magnitude of negative surface charge (Makino et al., 1991; Garcia-Manyes et al., 2006). The increased negative surface charge of invasomes prevents vesicle aggregation due to electrostatic repulsion, and thus ensures physical stability of invasomes (Dragicevic-Curic et al., 2008; Tawfik et al., 2020; El-Nabarawi et al., 2018). The addition of terpenes increased the negative surface charge of mTHPC-loaded invasomes to a small extent (Dragicevic-Curic et al., 2008), nimesulide-loaded invasomes to a higher extent (Badran et al., 2012), vardenafil-loaded ethosome-derived invasomes to a small extent, potentiating the effect of ethanol on the surface charge (Ammar et al., 2020).

The encapsulation efficiency (EE%) of drugs in invasomes is influenced by the type of terpene contained in invasomes. In the case of dapsone-loaded invasomes, the results showed that among the tested terpenes, limonene-containing invasomes showed the highest EE% of the lipophilic drug dapsone followed by cineole-, fenchone-, and citral-containing invasomes (El-Nabarawi et al., 2018). This could be attributed to the lipophilicity of the used terpenes (as manifested by their log P values, being 4.83, 2.82, 2.13, and 2.02 for limonene, cineole, fenchone, and citral, respectively). The higher the lipophilicity of the terpene, the higher the solubilization of the lipophilic drug, and hence the higher EE% owing to increased space for the drug incorporation in the lipid bilayer, resulting in high EE% (Mura et al., 2009). Thus, dapsone-loaded invasomes containing more lipophilic terpenes (limonene and cineole) possessed higher EE% compared to invasomes with less lipophilic terpenes (citral and fenchone). The same trend was seen for the drug EE% in agomelatine-loaded invasomes, being in the following descending order: limonene > cineole > fenchone > citral containing invasomes, and attributed to the lipophilicity of each terpene (Tawfik et al., 2020). This has been seen also for invasomes loaded with the highly lipophilic drug finasteride, where limonene and cineole-containing invasomes provided higher drug EE% than nerolidol-containing invasomes (Prasanthi et al., 2013). Invasomes containing the more lipophilic terpene limonene showed higher EE% of the highly lipophilic curcumin than invasomes containing the less lipophilic terpene fenchone (Lakshmi et al., 2014). Limonene-containing invasomes incorporating an antisense oligonucleotide drug exhibited higher drug EE% than invasomes containing cineole (Saffari et al., 2016). In addition to this, the use of eugenol increased the solubility and the entrapment of iso-tretinoin in invasomes (Dwivedi et al., 2017). Anastrozole being a hydrophilic drug has higher entrapment efficiency when combined with fenchone having lower lipophilicity (log P of fenchone = 2.13) (Vidya and Lakshmi, 2019).

In addition, the increase of terpene concentration in invasomes leads to an enhancement of the entrapment efficiency of drugs in invasomes, showing a direct relationship between terpene concentration and EE%. This was seen in the case of nimesulide-loaded invasomes (Badran et al., 2012), isotretinoin-loaded invasomes (Dwivedi et al., 2017), avanafil-loaded invasomes (Ahmed and Badr-Eldin, 2019), as well as in agomelatine-loaded invasomes upon increasing the terpene concentration from 0.75% w/v to 1.5% w/v (Tawfik et al., 2020), vardenafil hydrochloride invasomes increasing the terpene concentration from 0.55% w/v to 2% w/v (Ammar et al., 2020), etc. The enhanced EE% of drugs was attributed to the enhanced solubilization of drugs in the more lipophilic vesicles due to the increased concentration of the li-pophilic terpene in the phospholipid bilayers.

The EE% was also influenced by lecithin concentration in invasomes, i.e. the higher the amount of lecithin, the greater the tolterodine tartrate entrapment within the invasomes up to 3% lecithin, whereby a further increase in the concentration decreased the entrapment efficiency (Kalpana and Lakshmi, 2013). The increase in the entrapment efficiency with increasing phospholipid concentration was also seen in avanafil-, agomelatine- and isotretinoin-loaded invasomes and could be ascribed to the preferential localization of the drug in the lipid matrix (increasing with the increase of phospholipid concentration), rather than in the surrounding medium, due to its lipophilic nature (Tawfik et al., 2020; Dwivedi et al., 2017; Kamran et al., 2016).

Regarding the stability of liposomes, a lot of factors can influence the physical, as well as chemical stability, which is of high importance for drug safety (Thoma and Jocham, 1992). The storage temperature has a key role in the physical stability of invasomes, as an increase of the storage temperature from 4 °C to room temperature (RT) led to an increase in particle size and PDI value of mTHPC-loaded invasomes, especially in the case of higher terpene amounts. Thus, an increase of temperature, induced aggregation or fusion of vesicles. Namely, the mTHPC-loaded invasomes with 0.5% w/v terpenes were physically stable at 4 °C and room temperature (23 °C) during 12 months, since the size and PDI of vesicles did not change significantly. In contrast, the mTHPC-loaded invasomes containing 1% w/v terpenes were stable only when stored at 4 °C for 12 months (Figure 3.5). Thus, the addition of higher terpene amounts, i.e. 1% w/v terpenes, decreased the physical stability of vesicles when stored at room temperature (Dragicevic-Curic et al., 2008; Dragicevic-Curic et al., 2009). Higher stability at 4 °C was also seen for finasteride-loaded invasomes, as their vesicle size when stored at 4 °C did not vary, in contrast to their storage at 25 °C. The zeta potential and entrapment efficiency also changed, i.e. decreased when vesicles were stored at 25 °C (Prasanthi et al., 2013). Nimesulide-loaded invasomes revealed also physical stability when stored at 4 °C, as the particle size and the PDI of different nimesulide-loaded invasomes only slightly increased after 60 days of storage (Badran et al., 2012). As to the drug content in invasomes, the mTHPC-content did not change significantly during invasomes' storage (Dragicevic-Curic et al., 2008; Dragicevic-Curic et al., 2009). Thus, the recommendation is to store invasomes at 4 °C.

3.5 INVASOMES AS PENETRATION ENHANCERS

There is a vast number of studies confirming the ability of invasomes to enhance the percutaneous penetration of incorporated lipophilic or encapsulated

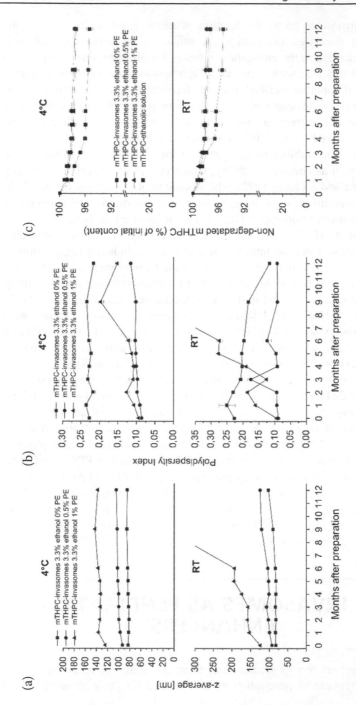

FIGURE 3.5 Stability study of mTHPC-liposomes containing 3.3% w/v ethanol and mTHPC-invasomes containing 0.5 and 1% w/v terpenes. (a) Change of the particle size of vesicles. (b) Change of the PDI of vesicles. (c) Change of the mTHPC-content in the different vesicles (Dragicevic-Curic et al., 2008).

hydrophilic drugs. Invasomes enable drug delivery to the deep skin layers as well as to the systemic circulation, thereby representing efficient dermal and transdermal drug delivery systems. In general, it has been shown that with increasing the amount of terpenes in invasomes, their penetration enhancing ability increases. However, the increase in terpene concentration is in direct correlation with the invasomes' particle size indicating a significant increase in particle size with the concentration of terpenes >1%. On the other hand, invasomes containing terpenes in concentration <1% possessed a lower penetration enhancement effect. Thus, a concentration of terpenes of 1% was taken as the optimum terpene concentration for most penetration studies. In this section, studies investigating the penetration enhancing ability of invasomes loaded with various drugs are discussed (Table 3.1).

3.5.1 Enhanced Percutaneous Penetration of Immunosuppresive Drugs

The first investigated invasomes were *cyclosporine A (CsA)*-loaded invasomes (Verma, 2002; Verma et al., 2003). CsA is an immunosuppressive drug used for the treatment of autoimmune diseases. It has been used in the management of psoriasis and other dermatological diseases that have inflammatory T-cell-mediated pathogenesis. Due to its stimulating effect on hair growth, it could be used for the treatment of alopecia areata and androgenetic alopecia. However, CsA is a lipophilic drug with a high molecular weight (MW) of 1202.61 Da and a partition coefficient (log P) of 2.9. Thus, CsA shows poor penetration into the skin, limiting its topical use. Therefore, invasomes were developed with the aim to enhance the percutaneous penetration of the drug CsA into the skin, as CsA does not possess favorable physicochemical properties to penetrate into the skin. CsA-loaded invasomes containing 10% w/v unsaturated soybean PC, 3.3% w/v ethanol, 0.5, 1.0 and 1.5% w/v of a terpene mixture composed of citral, cineole and d-limonene (cineole:citral:d-limonene = 45:45:10 v/v = standard terpene mixture) and phosphate buffer saline (PBS) up to 100% w/v were prepared (Verma, 2002). All invasomes provided *in vitro* in human skin significantly higher amounts of CsA in the deeper skin layers (viable epidermis and dermis) compared to conventional liquid-state liposomes (without ethanol and terpenes), and aqueous/ethanolic drug solution (Figure 3.6, Table 3.1). In addition, increasing the amount of terpenes from 0.5 to 1.5% increased the amount of CsA recovered in the SC and deeper skin layers, indicating a direct correlation between the amount of added terpenes and the amount of drug found in

TABLE 3.1 Invasomes as nanocarriers for dermal and transdermal drug delivery

FORMULATION	DRUG	INDICATION	CONDITION	OUTCOME	REF.
Invasomes 0.5–1.5% w/v terpene mixture (cineole:citral:d-limonene = 45:45:10 v/v)	Lipophilic drug Cyclosporine A (CsA)	Alopecia	In vitro human skin	Invasomes increased skin delivery of CsA compared to conventional liposomes and ethanolic solution. Increasing terpene concentration in invasomes increased skin deposition of mTHPC. Invasomes with 1.5% terpenes showed highest enhancing ability.	(Verma, 2002)
Invasomes 0.5–1% w/v terpene mixture (cineole:citral:d-limonene=45:45:10 v/v)	Hydrophobic drug Temoporfin (mTHPC)	Topical PDT	In vitro human skin	Invasomes increased skin delivery of mTHPC compared to conventional	(Dragicevic-Curic et al., 2008)

Invasomes with different terpenes/terpene mixtures 1% w/v d-limonene, 1% w/v citra 1%, w/v d-cineole Terpene mix = cineole:citral:d-limonene = 0.45:0.45:0.10 (v/v) = standard. Terpene mix1 = cineole:citral:d-limonene = 0.66:0.17:0.17 (v/v). Terpene mix2 = cineole:citral:d-limonene = 0.17:0.66:0.17 (v/v). Terpene mix3 = cineole:citral:d-	Hydrophobic drug Temoporfin (mTHPC)	Topical PDT	In vitro human skin	liposomes and ethanolic solution, whereby invasomes 1% terpenes showed highest penetration enhancing ability. iinvasomes 1% w/v citral provided the highest overall mTHPC-amount in the skin. Invasomes 1% w/v cineole delivered a high mTHPC-amount in the SC, and even into deeper skin layers.	(Dragicevic-Curic et al., 2009)

(Continued)

TABLE 3.1 (Continued) Invasomes as nanocarriers for dermal and transdermal drug delivery

FORMULATION	DRUG	INDICATION	CONDITION	OUTCOME	REF.
limonene = 0.17:0.17:0.66 (v/v). Terpene mix4 = cineole:citral:d-limonene = 0.33:0.33:0.33 (v/v). PEV 2% Transcutol® or Labrasol® or cineole	Minoxidil	Hair loss	In vitro new born pig skin	Labrasol®-PEVs and invasomes were approximately 3-folds more efficient than the control, while Transcutol®-PEVs enhanced only 1.3-fold the drug deposition in the SC compared to the control liposomes.	(Mura et al., 2009)

Invasomes 1% w/v terpene mixture (cineole:citral:d-limonene = 45:45:10 v/v), polysorbate 80-based liposomes, conventional liposomes and ethosomes	Amphiphilic drug Ferulic acid	Antioxidant activity	In vitro human SCE membrane	Ethosomes provided the highest skin flux and skin deposition of ferulic acid, being 75 times and 7.3 times higher than those obtained with saturated PBS (pH 7.4) solution, respectively.	(Chen et al., 2010)
Invasomes 1% w/v terpene mixture (cineole:citral:d-limonene = 45:45:10 v/v) and Core-multishell nanotransporters (CMS)	Hydrophilic spin label 2,2,5,5-tetramethyl-1-pyrrolidinyl-oxy-3-carboxylic acid (PCA)	Investigating the possibility to enhance the skin delivery of hydrophilic drugs	In vitro porcine ear skin	CMS delivered a 2.5-fold, invasomes delivered a 1.9-fold higher PCA amount to the skin than the solution.	(Haag et al., 2011)
nvasomes 1% w/v terpene mixture (cineole:citral:d-limonene = 45:45:10 v/v) Ethosomes	Hydrophilic dye carboxyfluorescein (CF)	Investigating the possibility to enhance the skin delivery of hydrophilic drugs	In vitro human skin	Invasomes and ethosomes improved the delivery of CF into the deep skin layers or across the skin.	(Chen et al., 2011)

(Continued)

TABLE 3.1 (Continued) Invasomes as nanocarriers for dermal and transdermal drug delivery

FORMULATION	DRUG	INDICATION	CONDITION	OUTCOME	REF.
Invasomes 1% terpenes (citral, limonene or cineole)	Nimesulide	Anti-inflammatory drug	In vitro, rat skin	Invasomes with 1% limonene provided highest cumulative drug amount permeated and highest drug flux.	(Badran et al., 2012)
Conventional liposomes, transfersomes, invasomes, aqueous solution	Hydrophilic dye Calcein	Investigating the possibility to enhance the skin delivery of hydrophilic drugs	In vitro human skin	Conventional liposomes enhanced *calcein* flux 1.2 times, transfersomes about 1.8 times, and invasomes 7.2 times compared to aqueous solution	(Ntimenou et al., 2012)
Invasomes containing different terpenes (limonene, fenchone, nerolidol: 0.5, 1.0, 1.5 %) and curcumin-HPβCD complex (5% w/v)	Curcumin	Antioxidant, antinflammatory agent	Ex vivorat skin	Invasomes with 0.5% limonene enhanced curcumin permeation by 8.11 times compared to the control.	(Lakshmi et al., 2014)

| Invasomes 0.5–3% terpene (limonene, cineole, fenchone, citral) | Dapsone | Antibacterial and anti-inflammatory activityTreatment of *Acne vulgaris* | Ex vivo, rat skinIn vivo, Wistar rats | Invasomes 1.5% limonene provided a 2.5-fold higher drug deposition in the skin than the drug solution. Gels incorporating invasomes containing 0.5 and 1% limonene provided a significantly higher drug flux than the control. | (El-Nabarawi et al., 2018) |
| Liposomes, invasomes, DDAB and CTAB LeciPlex | Azelaic acid Idebenone | Anti-acne drug Antioxidant (anticancer drug) | Ex vivo, human skinIn vivo, rats | LeciPlex increased delivery of idebenone whereas invasomes increased delivery of azelaic acid in ex vivo experiments. Azelaic acid invasomal gels showed the highest in vivo activity. | (Shah et al., 2015). |

(Continued)

TABLE 3.1 (Continued) Invasomes as nanocarriers for dermal and transdermal drug delivery

FORMULATION	DRUG	INDICATION	CONDITION	OUTCOME	REF.
Invasomes D-limonene and Cocamide diethanolamine	Capsaicin	Pain-relief	In vitroMice skin	Capsaicin-loaded invasomes exhibited higher skin permeability compared to conventional liposomes and the commercial product.	(Duangjit et al., 2016)
Invasomes Phospholipon®90G (6-12 w/v), β-citronellene (0.8–1.2% w/v) and ethanol (2-5% w/v)	Olmesartan	Antihypertensive drug	Ex vivo, rat skinIn vivo, Wistar rats	Optimized invasomes provided transdermal flux of 33 mg/cm^2/h. Invasomal gel showed a 1.15 times improvement in bioavailability of olmesartan with respect to the control marketed oral formulation	

Formulation	Drug	Indication	Skin model	Results	Reference
Ethosome-derived invasomes—limonene, cineole, mixture of limonene and cineole (1:1), at three concentrations (0.5%, 1% and 2%, v/v).	Vardenafil hydrochloride	Antihypertensive drug	Ex vivo, Wistar rat skin	Invasomes 1% terpene (0.5% limonene and 0.5% cineole) were the optimum formulation providing highest drug flux (ER = 15.5).	(Dwivedi et al., 2017)
Invasomes and invasomal gel	Isotretinoin	Eosinophilic pustular folliculitis	Ex vivo, rat skin	Invasomes provided cumulative drug permeation of 85.94% and a flux of approx. 78.82 µg/h/cm^2. Invasomal gel provided cumulative isotretinoin permeation within 8 h of 85.21%.	
Conventional liposomes cholesterol (0.5% w/v), soya PC (3% w/v);Invasomes d-limonene (1% w/v), 10% (v/v) ethanol,	Rezorcinol	Skin lightening agent	In vitro, pig skin	Liposomes, invasomes and transfersomes provided a cumulative drug amount	(Amnuaikit et al., 2018)

(Continued)

TABLE 3.1 (Continued) Invasomes as nanocarriers for dermal and transdermal drug delivery

FORMULATION	DRUG	INDICATION	CONDITION	OUTCOME	REF.
transfersomes sodium deoxycholate (15% w/ w related to lipid content)				permeated of 20.65, 47.99 and 72.66 µg/cm2, respectively, and a drug accumulation in the skin of 28.18, 54.43 and 71.21 µg/cm2, respectively.	
Invasomes PC (6, 10, 14 %), ethanol (2, 3.5, 5 %), terpene β-citronellol/limonene (1, 1.25, 1.5 %)	Avanafil	Phosphodiesterase type 5 (PDE5) inhibitor for treatment of erectile dysfunction	Ex vivo, Wistar rat skin, permeation study In vivo, Wistar rats, pharmacokinetic study	The enhancement ratio for cumulative amount of drug permeated from invasomal film was 2.514, relative to the raw avanafil film. A 4.5-fold increase in relative bioavailability was found for invasomal film compared to the raw AVA film.	

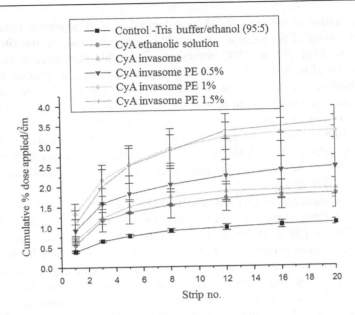

FIGURE 3.6 Skin penetration of cyclosporine A (CsA, CyA) after 6 h non-occlusive application of different CyA-formulations onto human abdominal skin (expressed as cumulative % of dose applied/cm^2 ±SE, n = 3). SC tape-stripping depth profile (Verma, 2002).

the skin. However, there was no statistically significant difference between invasomes containing 1% or 1.5% standard terpene mixture. This study proved the penetration enhancing ability of invasomes and revealed that invasomes present an effective carrier system for delivering the highly lipophilic CsA to the deeper skin layers where it should exert its therapeutic effect.

3.5.2 Enhanced Percutaneous Penetration of Photosensitizers

Since very promising results were obtained with CsA-loaded invasomes, these nanocarriers were also used to enhance the percutaneous penetration of the hydrophobic second-generation photosensitizer *temoporfin (mTHPC)*. The photosensitizer mTHPC is a candidate for topical photodynamic therapy (PDT) of cutaneous malignant and non-malignant diseases. Topical PDT with mTHPC would significantly simplify PDT compared to PDT after intravenous application of photosensitizers since in topical therapy the photosensitizer is directly applied onto the skin being readily accessible, the drug concentration in the skin would be enhanced as well as patient compliance and the residual photosensitivity would be restricted only to the site of application. However, mTHPC possesses unfavorable properties to easily penetrate the skin. It has a MW of 680 Da, and is highly hydrophobic (log P of 9.4 (Kelbauskas, 2003)). Consequently, mTHPC exhibits low percutaneous absorption and there are no topical formulations with mTHPC at the market. It has been to date applied only intravenously in PDT of skin cancers (Kübler et al., 1999). Thus, it was very important to use potent nanocarriers enabling the skin delivery of mTHPC, which would deliver sufficiently high amounts of mTHPC in the deeper skin layers to ensure a positive outcome of PDT of different skin diseases.

First studies were performed with mTHPC-loaded invasomes containing 0.5 and 1% w/v of the standard terpene mixture = cineole:citral:d-limonene = 45:45:10 v/v. Obtained results confirmed the ability of invasomes to enhance the percutaneous penetration of mTHPC. Invasomes were superior compared to conventional liposomes and other formulations, i.e., especially invasomes with 1% w/v terpene mixture represented a potent penetration enhancer (Figure 3.7,Table 3.1). Invasomes with 1% w/v terpene mixture delivered an approx. 3.5-, 2.7-, 2- and 1.7-fold higher mTHPC-amount to the SC than conventional liposomes, liposomes containing 3.3% w/v ethanol, ethanolic solution of mTHPC and invasomes containing 0.5% w/v terpenes, respectively. Invasomes with 1% w/v terpene mixture delivered mTHPC also into

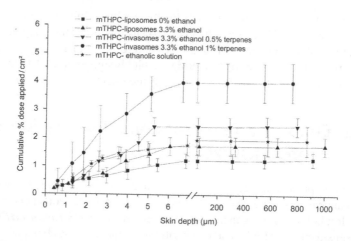

FIGURE 3.7 Skin penetration of mTHPC after 6 h non-occlusive application of different mTHPC-formulations onto human abdominal skin (expressed as cumulative % of dose applied/cm^2 ±SE, n = 3). Skin depth profile of mTHPC (Dragicevic-Curic et al., 2008).

the deeper skin layers (viable epidermis and dermis). However, as to deeper skin layers, they were only superior to the ethanolic solution of mTHPC. It was assumed that the mTHPC-amounts delivered to the SC and the deeper skin layers by all formulations, except the mTHPC-ethanolic solution, may be sufficient for an effective topical PDT (according to unpublished data from Biolitec AG, Germany). The highest total penetration enhancing effect was ascribed to mTHPC-loaded invasomes containing the highest amount of terpenes, i.e. 1% w/v standard terpene mixture. This was in accordance with the results obtained for CsA-loaded invasomes (Verma, 2002), showing a direct correlation between terpenes concentration and the amount of drug found in the skin.

In order to increase further the penetration enhancing ability of invasomes containing 1% w/v terpene mixture, the ratio between D-limonene, citral and cineole was varied in the standard terpene mixture and also single terpenes were used as additives (Dragicevic-Curic et al., 2009). As a result seven new mTHPC-loaded invasome dispersions were obtained, which were investigated for their penetration enhancing ability.

Obtained results revealed that dependent on the added terpene or terpene mixture, invasomes may enhance or retard the drug penetration into the skin compared to liposomes without terpenes. The addition of 1% w/v citral, 1% w/v cineole, or 1% w/v standard terpene mixture to liposomes containing 3.3% w/v ethanol resulted in the formation of highly effective skin delivery systems for mTHPC. Among these three formulations, invasomes with 1% w/v citral provided the highest overall mTHPC-amount in the skin, while invasomes with 1% w/v cineole provided a smaller total mTHPC-amount in the skin than invasomes with 1% w/v citral, but delivered besides the high mTHPC-amount in the SC, also a high mTHPC-amount in the deeper skin layers, representing therefore the optimal formulation (Table 3.1). Invasomes with 1% w/v standard terpene mixture provided high mTHPC-amounts in the SC and the deeper skin layers, but lower than invasomes with 1% w/v cineole. Thus, these three mTHPC-loaded invasome systems might be promising for the topical PDT of cutaneous disorders.

An interesting finding in this study was that invasomes containing high amounts of D-limonene in the terpene mixture or only D-limonene exhibited low enhancement ratios, which was unexpected. Limonene as a lipophilic terpene enhanced the skin delivery of the following lipophilic drugs: estradiol (Williams and Barry, 1991b), indomethacin (Ogiso et al., 1995), hydrocortisone (El-Kattan et al., 2001), midazolam (Ota et al., 2003) and others. The structure-activity relationship of terpenes was also confirmed by different authors (Hori et al., 1991; Moghimi et al., 1997), who found that hydrophilic terpenes (alcohols, ketones, and oxide terpenes, like fenchone and thymol) are more effective in enhancing the permeation of hydrophilic drugs (propranolol), while hydrocarbon terpenes (like limonene and cymene) are more effective in improving the permeation of lipophilic drugs (diazepam). The high lipophilicity of terpenes was thought to be an important property for enhancing the permeation of lipophilic drugs (Ghafourian et al., 2004). However, the addition of D-limonene failed to enhance the percutaneous penetration of mTHPC. This could be explained by the fact, that mTHPC cannot be considered as having a high affinity to the invasomal phospholipid membrane or the skin lipids (membrane-philic or highly lipophilic), but rather as a highly hydrophobic drug.

In contrast, the highest enhancement ratio of invasomes with 1% w/v citral, was not surprising, since citral is lipophilic and should therefore enhance the skin delivery of lipophilic substances (Williams and Barry, 1991a,b; Hori et al., 1991; Moghimi et al., 1997).

As to invasomes with 1% w/v cineole, the obtained results showing such high mTHPC-penetration into the SC and deeper skin layers were unexpected, since as aforementioned some studies showed that hydrophilic terpenes are less effective in enhancing the permeation of lipophilic drugs, and were ineffective in enhancing the permeation of the lipophilic drug indomethacin (Okabe et al., 1989). However, El-Kattan et al. (2001) showed that cineole provided among 12 different terpenes the highest amount of the lipophilic hydrocortisone in the skin, which would agree with the results obtained in this study. In addition, El-Kattan et al. reported that there was no correlation between the lipophilicity of terpenes and the amount of hydrocortisone in the skin (El-Kattan et al., 2001). The study with different terpene mixtures showed that besides the standard terpene mixture, also other terpene mixtures or single terpenes can be used to formulate invasomes possessing high penetration enhancing ability.

Anastrozole is an anti-cancer drug, i.e. a potent non-steroidal aromatase inhibitor, used for the management of postmenopausal women with breast cancer. However, anastrozole applied by the oral route shows many side effects and exhibits extensive first-pass metabolism. Since anastrozole possesses ideal properties required for transdermal delivery (log P = 3.5, MW = 293.3 Da, $t_{1/2}$ = 46.8 h), invasomes were used to encapsulate the drug and, thus, overcome its drawbacks. Anastrozole-loaded invasomes were composed of soya lecithin Phospholipon® 80H and soya PC Phospholipon® 90H (Lipoid AG), terpene (fenchone) and ethanol. Type of lipids, quantity of lipids, and percentage of terpene (2.5 and 4%) were varied. Optimized anastrozole-loaded invasomes containing 4% fenchone, being of sufficiently small particle size (226.4 nm), negative surface charge (-20.9 mV), providing highest skin deposition of the drug (11.18-fold higher compared to free drug) were further incorporated into a 5% sodium carboxymethyl cellulose (NaCMC) gel in order to obtain an invasomal gel. The *ex vivo* permeation and skin deposition revealed that invasomes showed superior permeation, enhanced transdermal flux, and 73% skin deposition of anastrozole. The highest *ex vivo* drug deposition in Wistar rat skin was found to be 149.2 µg/cm^2, provided by the invasomal gel compared to 24.33 µg/cm^2 and 31.39 µg/cm^2 provided by plain gels containing 2.5% and 4% terpene, respectively, followed by control gel depositing an amount of 11.38 µg/cm^2 (Table 3.1). Thus, the invasomal gel delivered a 13.11-fold higher anastrozole amount into the skin compared to the control gel (Vidya and Lakshmi, 2019).

3.5.3 Enhanced Percutaneous Penetration of Hydrophilic Model Drugs

Invasomes were able to enhance the penetration also of hydrophilic substances into the skin (Table 3.1). Namely, invasomes (5% w/v soybean PC, 10% v/v ethanol and 1% w/v standard terpene mixture) and core-multishell (CMS) nanotransporters were compared regarding their ability to enhance the skin delivery of the *hydrophilic spin label* 2,2,5,5-tetramethyl-1-pyrrolidinyl-oxy-3-carboxylic acid (*PCA*; log $P = -1.7$) (Haag et al., 2011). Electron paramagnetic resonance (EPR) spectroscopic techniques were used for the determination of the localization and distribution of the spin label within the nanocarriers and the ability of the nanocarriers to promote penetration of PCA into the skin. It has been shown that PCA was localized in the hydrophilic compartments of the nanocarriers. The *in vitro* study in porcine ear skin revealed that CMS nanotransporters provided higher amounts of the agent in the upper layers of the SC, whereas invasomes delivered the agent into the deeper SC layers (Figure 3.8). Moreover, compared to the solution of PCA, CMS nanotransporters delivered a 2.5-fold, while invasomes delivered 1.9-fold higher PCA amount to the skin. Invasomes provided PCA penetration enhancement which is in accordance with the results obtained for mTHPC-loaded invasomes compared to the mTHPC ethanolic solution (Dragicevic-Curic et al., 2008). The penetration of PCA applied in CMS nanocarriers agrees with the 2-fold enhanced penetration of the hydrophilic dye rhodamine B from CMS nanocarriers into the SC and epidermis of porcine skin compared to a base cream. The higher overall penetration enhancing effect of CMS nanocarriers compared to invasomes can be explained by the size of the carriers. The invasomes had a mean size of 190 nm, while the CMS nanocarriers possessed a mean size of 5 nm and thus could penetrate more easily into the superficial layers of the SC (Korting and Schäfer-Korting, 2010).

Moreover, Chen et al., (2011) reported that invasomes with 1% w/v terpene mixture (cineole:citral:d-limonene = 45:45:10 v/v) and ethosomes, regardless if

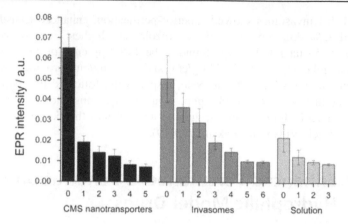

FIGURE 3.8   Spin label intensity of tape stripped porcine skin 30 min after application of PCA formulations. Tape number 0 corresponds to the intensity after penetration and removal of remaining liquids, number 1–6 correspond to the PCA related signal intensity of the skin after each tape strip taken. Mean ± SEM (n = 3) (Haag et al., 2011).

they were applied in finite (10 μl/cm²) or infinite doses (160 μl/cm²) *in vitro* in human skin, significantly improved the delivery of the *hydrophilic dye carboxyfluorescein (CF)* into the deep layers of the skin or across the skin compared to non-vesicular systems (solution in phosphate buffer, hydroethanolic solution). In contrast, the authors showed that in the case of mTHPC applied in finite or infinite dose, most of the drug was accumulated in the superficial skin layers (no mTHPC was detected in the dermis or the receptor phase), regardless if vesicular systems or non-vesicular systems were applied. Thus, the results suggested that lipid vesicles are more effective in improving the permeation and deposition of hydrophilic drugs such as CF than lipophilic drugs such as mTHPC (Chen et al., 2011).

As to the *hydrophilic dye calcein*, it was encapsulated into different vesicles, i.e. conventional liposomes, transfersomes with 1.1% sodium-cholate, and invasomes containing 1% of the standard terpene mixture. Permeation studies performed *in vitro* in human skin revealed that conventional liposomes enhanced calcein flux 1.2 times, transfersomes about 1.8 times, and invasomes 7.2 times compared to the calcein aqueous solution (Ntimenou et al., 2012). The drug flux and elasticity values for vesicles were correlated by rank order but not linearly, indicating that elasticity can be used only as a crude predictive tool to evaluate the potential of vesicles to enhance the penetration of the hydrophilic drug through the skin. Hence, other vesicle-related properties besides' elasticity may also influence the penetration enhancing ability of vesicles. Since the cumulative calcein amount (calcein permeated up to 10 h) provided by vesicles was not significantly different among the different elastic vesicles investigated, the authors assumed that it was possible for penetration enhancers to diffuse out from invasomes and permeate through the skin lipids to enhance drug transport. Thus, not only vesicle elasticity, but also other factors influence the transport of hydrophilic drug molecules through the skin (Ntimenou et al., 2012). Drug encapsulation efficiency was not found to be an important factor influencing drug penetration into the skin, since transfersomes were found to encapsulate almost a double amount of calcein, compared to invasomes.

3.5.4 Enhanced Percutaneous Penetration of Skin Lighteners

Phenylethyl resorcinol (4-(1-phenylethyl) 1, 3-benzenediol) is a new skin lightening agent, which inhibits the tyrosinase activity, even 22 folds more effectively than kojic acid (Chang, 2009). However, it possess poor aqueous solubility, low photostability and causes skin irritation, which limits its dermal use. To overcome these limitations, as well as to enhance its dermal delivery, phenylethyl resorcinol was incorporated into invasomes and transfersomes. The invasome formulations used fenchone, citral and D-limonene mixed with 10% (v/v) ethanol as skin enhancers. The liposomes were composed of 0.5% (w/v) CHOL, 3% (w/v) SPC and water up to 100% (v/v), whereas invasomes contained as a penetration enhancer additionally 0.5 to 1.5% w/v of a single terpene (fenchone, citral or D-limonene) mixed with 10% (v/v) ethanol, while transfersomes contained 5-15% w/w of Tween® 80, Tween® 20, Span® 80, Span® 20 or sodium deoxycholate as a penetration enhancer (Amnuaikit et al., 2018). Invasomes containing 1% (w/v) D-limonene and 10% (v/v) ethanol and transfersomes containing 15% (w/w) sodium deoxycholate were chosen as optimal formulations, being unilamellar (invasomes) or unilamellar to multilamellar (transfersomes), of spherical shape, with vesicle size approximately 350 nm, PDI <0.2, high zeta potential (42 and 60 mV, respectively), high EE% (approximately 90%), and good stability during storage at 30 °C at 75% RH for 4 months. Invasomes showed the highest deformability among vesicles, followed by transfersomes, while liposomes were rigid. This affected the *in vitro* skin permeation in newborn pig skin, as deformable vesicles provided a significantly higher cumulative amount, steady-state flux, and permeability coefficient compared to conventional liposomes. Liposomes, invasomes, and transfersomes provided a cumulative drug amount permeated of 20.65 ± 1.72 µg/cm^2, 47.99 ± 3.73 and 72.66 ± 4.66 µg/cm^2, respectively, and a cumulative drug amount in the skin of 28.18 ± 2.59, 54.43 ± 4.62 and 71.21 ± 8.40 µg/cm^2, respectively. Thus, invasomes were a more potent penetration enhancer than liposomes, however, transfersomes delivered the highest drug amounts into and through the skin.

3.5.5 Enhanced Percutaneous Penetration of Antioxidants

In an attempt to develop a suitable vesicular system for the dermal/transdermal delivery of the *amphiphilic drug ferulic acid* different vesicular systems were developed (Chen et al., 2010). Ferulic acid is a potent antioxidant with a variety of therapeutic effects, thereby being used in the treatment of skin diseases, diabetes, cardiovascular diseases, inflammatory disease, etc. Recently, it has started to be applied by injection, infusion, and perorally to treat cardiovascular diseases. However, due to the disadvantages of these administration routes (e.g. short elimination half-life after intravenous or intragastric administration, etc.), transdermal delivery of ferulic acid would be advantageous. Thus, invasomes with 1% w/v terpene mixture (cineole:citral:d-limonene = 45:45:10 v/v), polysorbate 80 (Tween® 80)-based deformable vesicles, conventional liposomes, and ethosomes (two formulations containing two different drug amounts) were investigated in terms of enhancing the percutaneous penetration of ferulic acid. All liposomal vesicles were of spherical shape, unilamellar in structure, of small particle size (<150 nm), high homogeneity (PDI <0.2) and negatively charged (except conventional liposomes). Results of *in vitro* skin permeation and skin deposition studies revealed that the permeation profile of ferulic acid through human stratum corneum/epidermis (SCE) membrane and the drug accumulation in the skin were both improved significantly using all vesicular systems, i.e. ethosomes, invasomes, transfersomes, and conventional liposomes compared to PBS solution of ferulic acid (Table 3.1) (Chen et al., 2010). Among all vesicles, ethosomes (with higher drug content) provided the highest skin flux and deposition of ferulic acid in the skin, being 75 times and 7.3 times higher than those obtained with saturated PBS (pH 7.4) solution, respectively. The deposited drug amount in the skin was far above the minimal effective concentration for e.g. an antioxidant effect of ferulic acid, while the obtained flux through the skin may be sufficient for achieving systemic drug effects.

3.5.6 Enhanced Percutaneous Penetration of Drugs for the Management of Prostatic Hyperplasia

Finasteride is a lipophilic 5-reductase inhibitor responsible for converting testosterone to active dihydrotestosterone. It is used in the treatment of benign prostatic hyperplasia and male pattern baldness (Alopecia). Finasteride has been used in the form of tablets. However, due to its low molecular weight 372.6 Da, half-life (6 h in individuals < 60 years old), bioavailability (63%), and log P (3.03), it represents a good candidate for transdermal drug delivery. Finasteride-loaded invasomes containing soya PC (10% w/v), different terpenes in various concentrations (limonene, carvone and nerolidol; 0.5, 1, 1.5% w/v) were developed using Taguchi robust design for optimization (Prasanthi et al., 2013). As to the factors affecting drug permeation *in vitro* in Wistar rat skin, the terpene type did not influence the cumulative drug amount permeated, whereas the concentration of terpenes had a significant effect on the cumulative drug amount permeated through the skin. The cumulative drug amount permeated through the skin was the least when invasomes containing 1.5% terpenes were used. Thus, invasomes with lower terpene concentrations were used (Table 3.1). Among invasomes with 1% terpenes, the highest drug permeation was achieved with invasomes containing 1% carvone (514.08 $\mu g/cm^2$) and nerolidol (503.05 $\mu g/cm^2$). As to limonene, invasomes containing 0.5% limonene showed maximum drug permeation (592.83 $\mu g/cm^2$). Invasomes containing 0.5% of the lipophilic terpene limonene enhanced the drug flux by 21.17 fold (22.8 $\mu g/cm^2/h$) when compared to control aqueous solution (1.08 $\mu g/cm^2/h$), thus, exhibiting the highest penetration enhancement of finasteride. It has already been reported that lipophilic limonene is able to enhance the permeation of a variety of hydrophobic drugs (Chen et al., 2016). This formulation has been used to further enhance the permeation of finasteride by iontophoresis (current density and pulse on/off ratio were optimized). Invasomes with 0.5% limonene applied together with iontophoresis (0.5 mA/cm^2, 3:1 pulse on/off ratio) enhanced drug flux by 25.83 fold when compared to control aqueous solution. This formulation combined with iontophoresis was further used in the form of a gel in an *in vivo* study in rabbits and compared to an oral drug suspension (Prasanthi et al., 2013). Pharmacokinetic parameters C_{max}, T_{max}, and the area under the curve (AUC) were calculated. AUC_{0-72h} and $T_{1/2}$ were 3.03- and 1.34-fold increased, respectively, when the invasomal gel of finasteride was used (as hepatic metabolism was reduced), showing an effective transdermal drug delivery, while C_{max} was lower after transdermal drug delivery. High C_{max} value upon oral administration was due to rapid absorption from the gastrointestinal tract, while low

C_{max} value obtained with transdermal gel can be attributed to the barrier property of the skin which leads to the accumulation of the drug in the skin and sustained release into the systemic circulation, which was shown by a 3- to 4-fold increase in AUC upon transdermal drug administration compared to oral administration. Overall, relative bioavailability of 303% was obtained with the invasomal gel compared to oral drug administration. The pharmacokinetic parameters confirmed a synergistic effect of invasomes and iontophoresis. Histopathological studies of the rat skin after the application of the invasomal gel revealed changes in the dermis indicating an effect of ethanol and terpenes present in invasomes. Application of iontophoresis showed severe irritation effects. On the basis of all results, invasomes represent effective drug nanocarriers for iontophoretic transdermal delivery of finasteride (Prasanthi et al., 2013).

Invasomes were also used as nanocarriers of *tolterodine tartrate* applied in the treatment of overactive bladder with the aim to develop a transdermal drug delivery system, as oral administration of tolterodine tartrate shows a lot of adverse side effects (e.g. dry mouth, tachycardia, dizziness, and gastrointestinal obstructive disorder). This was achievable since tolterodine tartrate has the ideal characteristics for transdermal drug delivery, such as low application dose < 10 mg/day, aqueous solubility >1 mg/ml, log P between 1 and 3, MW < 500 Da, and half life < 10 h. Tolterodine tartrate-loaded invasomes were prepared using soya lecithin (1, 3, 5, and 7%), ethanol (10% v/v), and three different terpenes (1% v/v, limonene, fenchone, and anethole). Invasomes containing 1% terpenes with the highest entrapment efficiency (containing 3% PC) were further investigated for their penetration enhancing effect *ex vivo* in Wistar rat skin, revealing their superiority in enhancing percutaneous penetration of the drug over vesicles without terpenes, ethanolic drug solution and aqueous drug solution (Table 3.1). The order of permeation enhancement was the following invasomes 1% limonene > invasomes 1% anethole > invasomes 1% fenchone, thus limonene with highest lipophilicity provided the highest increase in flux of the slightly lipophillic drug, while fenchone with lowest lipophilicity provided the lowest drug flux. The high penetration enhancing effect of limonene could be explained by earlier findings that lipophilic terpenes encapsulated in invasomes enhance permeation of both hydrophilic and lipophilic drugs (Dragicevic-Curic et al., 2009; Chen et al., 2011). Further, the authors ascribed this higher penetration enhancing effect of limonene to its low boiling point, as the low boiling point of terpenes indicate weak cohesiveness or self-association of the molecules and therefore they may more easily associate or interact with lipid components of the SC and alter their barrier property (Kalpana and Lakshmi, 2013). Invasomes containing 1% limonene being the most efficient formulation provided an enhanced penetration and accumulation of tolterodine tartrate in the skin compared to the vesicles without terpenes. However, a significantly enhanced permeation by invasomes with 1% limonene, being 3.4 fold higher, was observed when compared to the drug solution. In order to further enhance the drug permeation iontophoresis was used alone or combined with invasomes. Invasomes were superior to iontophoresis, when both were used as single methods. However, when iontophoresis was used together with invasomes, an additive effect of applied methods on the flux of tolterodine tartrate was observed. The flux increased from 0.0086 to 0.0135, when invasomes with limonene or iontophoresis were used alone, to 0.0387 $\mu g/h/cm^2$, respectively, when methods were combined. As to invasomes and the drug solution, iontophoretic drug transport showed that the permeability of tolterodine tartrate released from invasomes was higher compared to that of the free drug, also confirming the additive effect of invasomes and iontophoresis (Kalpana and Lakshmi, 2013). Thus, the combination of invasomes as a chemical method and iontophoresis as a physical method provided higher transdermal drug delivery compared to the use of single enhancement methods.

3.5.7 Enhanced Percutaneous Penetration of Curcumin

Curcumin is a yellow polyphenol obtained from rhizomes of *Curcuma longa lin*. It shows antioxidant, antiinflammatory, anticarcinogenic, hypocholesterolemic, antibacterial, antispasmodic, anticoagulant, antitumor, and other effects. However, it has poor aqueous solubility, low systemic bioavailability, exhibits photodegradation, etc. Lakshmi et al. (2014) developed, therefore, curcumin-loaded invasomes to overcome these disadvantages. Firstly, they increased the solubility of curcumin by complexing it with cyclodextrin (CD) and hydroxy propyl β-cyclodextrin (HPβCD), by physical mixture or the co-precipitation method. The complex with HPβCD in 1:2 proportion obtained by co-precipitation was found to bind 90% of curcumin. Afterwards the authors incorporated this complex into invasomes, being further converted to an invasomal gel by adding them into a 2% HPMC gel. Invasomes were composed of SPC (1% w/v), different terpenes (limonene, fenchone, nerolidol: 0.5, 1.0, 1.5 %), curcumin-HPβCD complex (5% w/v), ethanol (4% w/v) and PBS up to 100% w/v (Lakshmi et al., 2014). Three invasome formulations showing a good release rate were selected for *ex vivo* permeation studies in rat skin. Invasomes with 0.5% limonene, invasomes with 1% limonene and invasomes with 1% fenchone provided cumulative drug amounts permeated (Q_{24}) of approximately 70.32 $\mu g/cm^2$, 60.58 $\mu g/cm^2$, 51.8 $\mu g/cm^2$, respectively, being significantly higher than that of conventional liposomes, i.e. 22.89 $\mu g/cm^2$. This finding was attributed to the synergistic effect of ethanol and terpenes as liposomal formulation prepared without terpenes also showed an increase in permeation of 40.32 μg/cm^2, however lower than invasomes. As to the transdermal drug flux, conventional liposomes provided a flux of 0.41 μg/cm^2/h, while maximum flux was observed for curcumin-loaded invasomes containing 0.5% limonene and 4% ethanol, being significantly higher, i.e. 3.34 μg/cm^2/h. Thus, invasomes with 0.5% limonene enhanced curcumin permeation by 8.11 times compared to the control (Table 3.1). These results were in accordance with El-Kattan et al. (2001), where limonene showed a high penetration enhancing effect regarding lipophilic drugs. The permeation enhancement obtained with invasomes containing limonene may be due to its lipophilicity and low boiling point (Kalpana and Lakshmi, 2013) and the lipophilic nature of curcumin. Invasomes with 0.5% and 1% limonene were incorporated into the gel and the *ex vivo* permeation study revealed that these gels provided cumulative drug amount permeated of 52.8 μg/cm^2 and 42.32 μg/cm^2, respectively, while the control provided a cumulative drug amount of 7.98 μg/cm^2. As to the steady state transdermal flux, it was found to be 2.21 and 1.77 μg/cm^2/h for gels incorporating invasomes containing 0.5 and 1% limonene, respectively, and 0.28 μg/cm^2/h for the control, being significantly lower. The authors confirmed the ability to enhance curcumin solubility by complexing it with HPβCD, as well as the ability of the invasomal gel with 0.5% limonene to significantly enhance the percutaneous penetration of curcumin compared to the control (Lakshmi et al., 2014).

As to curcumin-loaded invasomes, Duangjit et al. developed different vesicles containing penetration enhancers (limonene, Tween® 20) (Duangjit et al., 2016). The authors investigated the effect of the penetration enhancers contained in invasomes and flexosomes (containing only Tween® 20) on the intercellular SC lipids by FTIR and DSC. The results confirmed that the penetration enhancers increased the fluidity of the skin lipids, as they decreased the transition temperature of the intercellular skin lipids. This phenomenon would enable enhanced curcumin penetration through the fluidized skin lipids.

3.5.8 Enhanced Percutaneous Penetration of Antihypertensive Drugs

As a large number of antihypertensive drugs used by the oral route undergo extensive first-pass metabolism, have low oral bioavailability, and other disadvantages, transdermal drug delivery would be advantageous as it circumvents adverse reactions and inconveniences linked to the oral route.

Transdermal drug delivery systems deliver drugs at a predetermined and controlled rate (Ahad et al., 2015), which is particularly desired in the treatment of chronic disorders, like hypertension (Ahad et al., 2013). Therefore, Qadri et al. (2017) developed invasomes loaded with the lipophilic drug *isradipine*, being an effective calcium channel blocker used in the management of hypertension. Isradipine-loaded invasomes were composed of soya lecithin, i.e. Phospholipon®90 G (Lipoid AG) (1–3% w/v), β-citronellene (0.1–0.5% w/v) and ethanol (10% w/v). The optimal isradipine-loaded invasomes (2% Phospholipon®90G, 0.1% β-citronellene, 10% ethanol), being of low particle size (194 nm), high entrapment efficiency (88.46%), enhanced drug flux *in vitro* through rat skin, providing a mean transdermal flux of 22.80 mg/cm^2/h. CLSM revealed an enhanced permeation of Rhodamine-Red-loaded isradipine invasomes to the deeper layers of the rat skin (approximately to 171 μm skin depth). Thus, invasomes enhanced the delivery of isradipine in terms of depth and quantity (Table 3.1). They, showed also high therapeutic effectiveness *in vivo* in Wistar rats (see Section 3.7.4).

Olmesartan is also a hydrophobic antihypertensive drug with a short biological half-life, and low oral bioavailability, thus, being a good candidate for transdermal drug delivery. Therefore, Kamran et al. (2016) developed and optimized using the Box-Behnken design olmesartan-loaded invasomes containing β-citronellene, as a membrane modifier inducing deformability to vesicles' bilayers and as a potential penetration enhancer. Olmesartan-loaded invasomes were composed of Phospholipon®90G (6-12 w/v), β-citronellene (0.8–1.2% w/v) and ethanol (2–5% w/v). The terpene concentration and phospholipid content were directly proportional to the vesicle size and entrapment efficiency. Further, the transdermal flux of olmesartan increased with increasing the phospholipid concentration in the formulation, as well with β-citronellene concentration, which was in accordance with previous findings obtained for CsA-loaded and mTHPC-loaded invasomes (Dragicevic-Curic et al., 2008; Verma, 2002). However, invasomes with the following composition: phospholipid (11.11 mg), ethanol (4.35%), and β-citronellene (1.09%) were found to be the optimal olmesartan invasomes. These optimal invasomes possessed a vesicle size of 83 nm, entrapment efficiency of 65 %, and provided a transdermal flux of 33 mg/cm^2/h. These experimental values were in agreement with the predicted value of vesicles size (94.69 nm), entrapment efficiency (68.47%) and transdermal flux (30.69 mg/cm^2/h) generated by Design Expert software®. CLSM of rat skin showed that optimized invasomes were eventually distributed and permeated deep into the skin as fluorescence intensity was high and seen up to about 168 μm skin depth. This efficient delivery of Rhodamine B marker by invasomes suggested that invasomes were able to penetrate into deeper skin layers where they fuse with the intercellular lipids, which would be in accordance with the hypothesis of many researchers (Ainbinder et al., 2016; Touitou et al., 2000; Chourasia et al., 2011; Sharma et al., 2014). This can be attributed to the high penetration enhancing capacity of β-citronellene, as it has been identified as a potent penetration enhancer for transdermal delivery of hydrophilic and lipophilic drugs (e.g. valsartan) possibly due to its melting point (154–155 °C) and log P (5.012) (Aqil et al., 2007; Ahad et al., 2011; Ahad et al., 2011; Ahad et al., 2009).

The pharmacokinetic study performed *in vivo* in Wistar rats revealed that C_{max} achieved by the application of invasomes was significantly ($p < 0.05$) lower than that of the oral tablets, however the AUC values were significantly higher ($p < 0.05$). The significantly high AUC_{0-48} value (3839 ng·h/ml) obtained with olmesartan-loaded invasomes compared to that obtained after oral administration (3320.99 ng·h/ml) indicates increased bioavailability of the drug from the transdermal route as compared to the oral route, which was probably due to the avoidance of hepatic metabolism. It also shows maintenance of the drug concentration within the pharmacologically effective range for a longer period of time. Overall, the relative bioavailability AUC transdermal/AUC oral was calculated to be 115.60%. Thus, the optimized invasomal gel showed a 1.15 times improvement in bioavailability of olmesartan with respect to the control marketed oral formulation. The authors confirmed that transdermal olmesartan delivery by invasomes as drug carriers offers a better alternative to the oral drug administration, exhibiting higher bioavailability and lesser dose frequency for the antihypertensive drug olmesartan (Kamran et al., 2016).

Vardenafil hydrochloride is a phosphodiesterase-5 (PDE-5) inhibitor used in the management of pulmonary arterial hypertension (PAH) and is more potent in inhibiting PDE-5 than sildenafil or tadalafil (Ammar et al., 2020). However, the therapeutic efficiency of vardenafil following oral administration is limited due to its low aqueous solubility (0.11 mg/mL), short biological half-life (≈ 4–5 h) and limited oral bioavailability (15%), as it undergoes hepatic first-pass metabolism. Thus, vardenafil is a candidate for transdermal drug delivery since this route of drug administration would circumvent the mentioned disadvantages of the oral drug administration, thereby enhancing drug bioavailability. Amar *et al.* developed and optimized vardenafil-loaded ethosome-derived invasomes in order to enable transdermal delivery of vardenafil. The authors developed firstly vardenafil-loaded ethosomes of different PC (5, 15 and 25 mg/mL) and ethanol (20%, 30% and 40%, v/v) concentration. All obtained ethosomes were of small particle size (138–198 nm), narrow size distribution (PDI = 0.174–0.258), high EE% (from 70.5% to 77.7%), and negative surface charge (ranging from −6.34 mV to 0.8 mV). Ethosomes with the highest PC and ethanol amount were of the smallest particle size, highest negative surface charge, and highest EE% (due to the fact that PC forms strong coherent bilayers preventing drug escape and ethanol enhances the solubility of vardenafil). As to *ex vivo* permeation studies performed in Wistar rats, they revealed a direct correlation between PC concentration and drug permeation, at a constant ethanol concentration, as well as between ethanol concentration and drug permeation, at a constant PC concentration, which was expected due to the penetration enhancing effects of PC and ethanol. The highest flux of 3.1 $\mu g \cdot cm^{-2} \ h^{-1}$ and consequently the highest enhancement ratio (15.5) was achieved by the aforementioned ethosome formulation, which was further optimized by the incorporation of terpenes (limonene, cineole, mixture of limonene and cineole in ratio 1:1) at three concentrations (0.5%, 1% and 2%, v/v). As to the penetration enhancing ability obtained invasomes showed superiority compared to ethosomes, as the flux values ranged from 3.2 $\mu g \cdot cm^{-2} \ h^{-1}$ (for invasomes 0.5% limonene) to 6.4 $\mu g \cdot cm^{-2} \ h^{-1}$ (for invasomes 1% terpene, i.e. 0.5% limonene and 0.5% cineole; optimal invasomal formulation) (Table 3.1). In addition, systems containing mixtures of limonene and cineole provided higher flux values compared to invasomes containing either cineole or limonene. The optimal invasomes were of a spherical size, small vesicle size (159.9 nm), possessing negative zeta potential (−20.3 mV), high EE% (81.3%), low $Q_{0.5h}$ (25.4%), high Q_{12h} (85.3%), and provided the largest steady-state flux (6.4 $\mu g \cdot cm^{-2} \ h^{-1}$) and enhancement ratio of 15.5 compared to the aqueous drug dispersion. CLSM studies with rhodamine B proved their ability to deeply permeate rat skin as the invasomes were deposited over the SC, the epidermis and the hypodermis layers with higher fluorescence intensities. The driving force for enhancing drug permeation through the skin was attributed to the synergistic effect of PC, ethanol, and terpenes. The authors proposed, three skin permeation pathways for the drug, through corneocytes as a transcellular route, between corneocytes as a paracellular route, and through appendages. They support the theory of Dragicevic-Curic et al. (2008), that some invasomes might break up during permeation in the upper skin layers, thus releasing ethanol, terpenes, and PC which fluidize the intercellular lipids, allowing the drug to permeate into deep skin layers. On the other hand, ethanol and terpenes contained in smaller invasomes can similarly fluidize vesicle bilayers, enhance their flexibility and permeation via the hair-follicles and/or the narrow hydrophilic channels distributed within the intercellular lipids. The apparent intense fluorescence near the hair follicles could be attributed to the localized accumulation of the developed lipophilic vesicles. Due to the authors, the follicular pathway could be described as the main skin permeation route for vardenafil-loaded invasomes, and it is expected that invasomes reach the systemic circulation as microreservoir systems able to sustain the rate of drug release and/or improve its bioavailability since blood capillaries surround the hair follicles (Shamma et al., 2019). The physiologically-based pharmacokinetic (PBPK) modeling revealed also an enhanced bioavailability of vardenafil following the transdermal application of invasomes in adults and geriatrics. Thus, vardenafil-loaded ethosome-derived invasomal systems represent a promising transdermal drug delivery system that could be used for the management of pulmonary arterial hypertension.

3.5.9 Enhanced Percutaneous Penetration of Isotretinoin for the Treatment of Eosinophilic Pustular Folliculitis

Isotretinoin is an analog of vitamin A (retinoid), which alters the DNA transcription mechanism and interferes in the process of DNA formation. It has been used in eosinophilic pustular folliculitis (Dwivedi et al., 2017). Dwivedi et al. (2017) prepared applying a 3^2 factorial design different isotretinoin-loaded invasomes with the aim to develop an isotretinoin-loaded invasomal gel able to deliver and target the drug to the pilosebaceous follicular unit. Among different invasomes, the optimal vesicles were those showing a small particle size of 148 nm, a low PDI value of 0.16, a high zeta potential of –69.2 mV, and a high entrapment efficiency of 85.78%. These invasomes showed *ex vivo* in rat skin a cumulative isotretinoin permeation of 85.94% and a flux of approximately 78.82 µg/h/cm^2 (Table 3.1) The optimal invasomes were further formulated into an invasomal gel, which provided a drug content of 97.12%, zero-order release kinetic with a 1.135 diffusion constant (Kd) and a cumulative isotretinoin permeation within 8 h of 85.21%. CLSM studies confirmed that invasomes from the invasomal gel successfully reached the pilosebaceous follicular unit. The invasomal gel was further studied in cell line SZ-95 and exhibited IC50 of ≤8 (at 25 µM of isotretinoin). Cell cycle analysis confirmed that the isotretinon-loaded invasomal gel inhibited the cell growth up to 82% with insignificant difference to pure isotretenion. Thus, the authors demonstrated that the invasomal gel was capable of delivering isotretinoin to the follicular unit, thereby providing pilosebaceous targeting.

3.5.10 Enhanced Percutaneous Penetration of Nonsteroidal Anti-Inflammatory Drugs

Invasomes were developed to incorporate and, hence, to improve the percutaneous penetration of the nonsteroidal anti-inflammatory drug (NSAID) *nimesulide* used here as a hydrophobic model drug, having very low water solubility (0.01 mg/mL), log P of 2.60 and a pKa value of 6.46 (Badran et al., 2012). Invasomes were composed of soybean lecithin 10%, ethanol 3.3% and 1% terpenes (citral, limonene or cineole). Badran et al. investigated the effect of the terpenes incorporated in invasomes on the *in vitro* skin delivery of nimesulide in abdominal rat skin in comparison to conventional liposomes and ethanolic drug solutions (Badran et al., 2012). All obtained invasomes were of spherical shape with negative zeta potential (from approx. −22.6 to −32.4 mV), low polydispersity (PDI < 0.2), small particle size (from 194.1 to 244.1 nm), high EE% (from 76.4 to 83.7%) and good physical stability. Results of the *in vitro* skin permeation study revealed that invasomes provided significantly higher drug permeation through rat skin compared with conventional liposomes and drug solution, while conventional liposomes were superior to the hydroethanolic solution. Thus, results showed that the improved permeation of nimesulide containing 1% terpenes (and 3.3% ethanol) was not only a result of the amount of terpenes, but also a result of the potential synergistic effect of ethanol and terpenes, which was in accordance with previous findings (Dragicevic-Curic et al., 2009). The drug permeation data obtained by different formulations were ranked in the following order: invasomes 1% limonene > invasomes 1% citral > invasomes 1% cineole > conventional liposomes > hydroethanolic solution, i.e., drug amounts in the receptor fluid obtained by invasomes containing 1% limonene were 18.09, 9.43, 7.10 and 2.16-fold higher compared to the hydroethanolic solution, conventional liposomes, invasomes containing cineol and citral, respectively. The flux of nimesulide was enhanced to 20.51 µg/cm^2/h with invasomes with 1% limonene (most potent invasomes), which was about 17.47, 8.60, 3.77 and 1.61 fold higher compared to the drug solution, conventional liposomes, invasomes 1% cineol and invasomes 1% citral, respectively. Invasomes with 1% limonene were able also to provide the highest cumulative percentage of nimesulide permeated through rat skin, approximately 29%, i.e. 869.708 µg, being 3.29-fold higher compared to that provided by invasomes with 1% cineol, being the least efficient invasomes. Thus, it was suggested that nimesulide skin delivery was strictly correlated to the type of terpenes incorporated into liposomes (Badran et al., 2012). This may be due to the fact that limonene has the highest log P (4.58), i.e., higher than citral (3.45) and cineol (2.82) (El-Kattan et al., 2000), whereby the efficiency of limonene had also been confirmed for transdermal delivery of ketoprofen, indomethacin and estradiol (Williams and Barry, 2004). Thus, invasomes with 1% limonene represent a promising nanocarrier for the transdermal delivery of the lipophilic drug nimesulide.

Capsaicin has been used for the management of oral and topical pain. However, its pungency and water insolubility restrict the use of capsaicin. In order to overcome these drawbacks, as well as to enhance its percutaneous penetration, capsaicin (0.15%) was encapsulated into invasomes, which contained besides PC and CHOL, various concentrations of D-limonene and cocamide diethanolamine (non-ionic surfactant). Optimum invasomes were estimated by the computer software (Design Expert®) and experimentally formulated and investigated. The optimized capsaicin-loaded invasomes were of small particle size (<100 nm), high homogeneity, and negative surface charge (−20mV). Further, capsaicin-loaded invasomes exhibited higher skin permeability compared to conventional liposomes and the commercial product, i.e., 0.15% capsaicin in ethanolic solution (Table 3.1) (Duangjit et al., 2016).

3.5.11 Enhanced Percutaneous Penetration of Drugs for the Treatment of *Acne Vulgaris*

Dapsone is a unique sulfone with antibiotic and anti-inflammatory activity, exhibiting therefore great potential to treat mild to moderate acne. Due to serious side effects of oral administration of dapsone, it has been proposed to apply dapsone topically onto the skin to reduce systemic exposure and alleviate associated side effects. El-Nabarawi et al. (2018) developed dapsone-loaded invasomes composed of PC, ethanol, and a single terpene or a mixture of terpenes (limonene, cineole, fenchone, and citral) used at different concentrations (0.5, 1.5 and 3%), for enhanced percutaneous drug permeation. The goal was to obtain an optimum dapsone-loaded invasome formulation with the highest EE%, lowest particle size, highest % of released dapsone after 2 and 24 h, and highest release efficiency. The optimum invasomes contained 1.5% limonene and their penetration enhancing ability was investigated *ex vivo* in rat skin and *in vivo* in Wistar rat skin. The amount of dapsone retained *ex vivo* in rat skin after the 24 h treatment with dapsone solution and invasomes was equivalent to 120.24 and 457.56 µg/mL, respectively, indicating an approximately 4-fold enhancement when using invasomes. Further, *in vivo* in Wistar rats invasomes provided an approximately 2.5-fold higher deposited amount of dapsone in the skin compared to the drug alcoholic solution, i.e. invasomes delivered a drug amount of 4.11 mcg/cm^2 compared to 1.71 mcg/cm^2 provided by the drug alcoholic solution (Figure 3.9). This result was expected as invasomes represent efficient penetration enhancers for hydrophobic drugs (Dragicevic-Curic et al., 2008). Further, the AUC_{0-10}

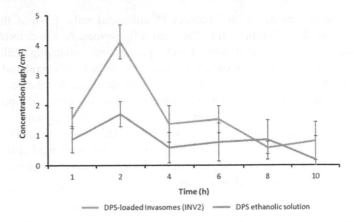

FIGURE 3.9 *In vivo* skin deposition profiles of dapsone (DPS) after topical treatment with DPS-loaded invasomes and DPS solution. INV2-invasomes with 1.5% limonene (El-Nabarawi et al., 2018).

calculated for dapsone-loaded invasomes was nearly 2-fold higher than that of the dapsone solution (14.54 and 8.01 mcg·h/cm², respectively) (El-Nabarawi et al., 2018). Thus, the authors showed that invasomes could enhance the skin accumulation of dapsone, thus, enabling the delivery of therapeutic drug amounts to the skin, which is a prerequisite for a positive outcome of the treatment of *Acne vulgaris*.

3.5.12 Enhanced Percutaneous Penetration of Drugs for the Treatment of *Alopecia*

Minoxidil used in the treatment of hair loss was encapsulated into different penetration-enhancer containing vesicles (PEV). PEVs were prepared by using soy lecithin and one of three penetration enhancers, 2-(2-ethoxyethoxy) ethanol (Transcutol®, Trc), capryl-caproyl macrogol 8-glyceride (Labrasol®, Lab), and cineole in order to enhance the skin penetration of minoxidil. All penetration enhancers were used at the same concentration (2%) (Mura et al., 2009). Penetration studies performed *in vitro* in new born pig skin showed no permeation of minoxidil through the skin regardless if PEVs were used or the control (conventional liposomes). In contrast, all PEVs enhanced the drug penetration into the skin compared to the control, while the highest drug amount was found in the SC (Table 3.1). Vesicles with Labrasol® and vesicles with cineole (invasomes) were approximately 3-folds more efficient than the control, while vesicles with Transcutol® enhanced only 1.3-fold the drug deposition in the SC compared to the control liposomes. As the deformability of vesicles has the crucial role in their penetration enhancing ability, the authors concluded that the penetration data were strictly correlated to vesicles deformability. Trc-PEVs were the least deformable vesicles among PEVs, i.e. they were only more deformable than conventional liposomes. Lab-PEVs and cineole-PEVs were 6- and 5-fold more elastic than conventional liposomes and 3- and 2-fold more deformable than Trc-PEVs, respectively. This was a consequence of the different chemical structure of the penetration enhancer, and thus different interaction with the phospholipid bilayers of vesicles (Mura et al., 2009).

3.5.13 Enhanced Percutaneous Penetration of Drugs for the Treatment of Erectile Dysfunction

Avanafil (AVA) is a novel selective phosphodiesterase type 5 (PDE5) inhibitor used for the treatment of erectile dysfunction. It is approved by FDA to be used via oral administration. However, avanafil suffers from poor aqueous solubility, considerable presystemic metabolism and altered absorption in the presence of food, and, thus, limited oral bioavailability. Therefore, transdermal drug delivery would be advantageous as it surmounts the GIT and its effects on the drug, as well as the first pass effect of drugs, besides other advantages (such as enhanced compliance due to painless administration compared to invasive routes of application, controlled drug delivery, reduced side effects, etc.). However, the main obstacle for transdermal delivery is the reduced penetration of drugs through the SC exerting barrier property. Thus, invasomes were used to circumvent the unfavorable properties of avanafil (molecular weight of 483.951 g/mol, two pKa values, 11.84 [acidic] and 5.89 [basic], log P value = 1.84, low solubility in water, methanol, and ethanol [< 1 mg/mL at 25 °C]), as well as to enable its transdermal delivery (Ahmed and Badr-Eldin, 2019). Avanafil-loaded invasomes were prepared and the influence of different concentrations of phospholipid (6, 10, 14%), ethanol (2, 3.5, 5%), terpene (1, 1.25, 1.5%), and terpene type (β-citronellol and limonene) on vesicle size and high entrapment efficiency (according to a Box-Behnken experimental design) were investigated. The authors found that the optimal invasomes formulation was composed of 10.47% phospholipid, 2% (ethanol), 1.5% D-limonene, showing a small vesicle size of 109.92 nm and entrapment efficiency of 96.98%. This

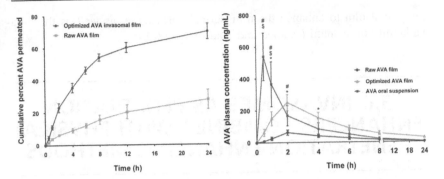

FIGURE 3.10 (A) Mean cumulative avanafil (AVA) percentage permeated across excised rat abdominal skin from optimized AVA invasomal film compared to raw AVA film. (B) AVA plasma concentration-time plot following application of AVA invasomal transdermal film, raw AVA transdermal film and AVA suspension (administered orally). Data represent the mean value ± standard deviation (SD), n = 12. #Significant at $P < 0.05$, for AVA oral suspension vs raw AVA transdermal films. $ Significant at $P < 0.05$, for optimized AVA invasomal transdermal film vs AVA oral suspension (Ahmed and Badr-Eldin, 2019).

formulation was further incorporated into a hydroxypropylmethyl cellulose (2% v/w)-based transdermal film in order to obtain avanafil invasomal films. These invasomal films were investigated *ex vivo* in abdominal Wistar rat skin for their permeation behavior and compared to raw avanafil films. The results showed that invasomal films provided a significantly higher cumulative percentage of drug permeated, as well as higher permeability and diffusion coefficients compared to the raw avanafil films. The enhancement ratio for a cumulative amount of drug permeated from the optimized invasomal film was 2.514 relative to the raw avanafil film (Figure 3.10). The pharmacokinetic assessment of avanafil invasomal films was carried out *in vivo* in Wistar rats, and a more than four-fold increase (451.44%) in relative bioavailability was found compared to the raw AVA film (Figure 3.10). However, the invasomal film demonstrated a significantly higher AUC and a relative bioavailability of 148.5% compared even to the oral suspension. The increased bioavailability from the invasomal transdermal film could be due to circumventing the presystemic metabolism of the drug, while the lower C_{max} and longer T_{max} obtained by the invasomal film compared to the oral suspension might be due to the invasomes' ability to control drug release and consequently its absorption. These results demonstrated once more the superiority of invasomal formulations, whereby here confirming the capability of the avanafil-loaded

invasomal film to enhance the transdermal permeation, as well as the bioavailability of avanafil (Ahmed and Badr-Eldin, 2019).

3.6 INVASOMES AS PENETRATION ENHANCERS COMBINED WITH PHYSICAL PENETRATION ENHANCING METHODS

The use of nanocarriers is generally mainly confined to achieving dermal
delivery of drugs, while transdermal drug delivery can be achieved, but less
frequent than the dermal drug delivery. However, nanocarriers as a chemical
penetration enhancement method are often combined with another penetration
enhancement method, especially with one of the physical methods. These two
methods enhance drug penetration via different enhancement mechanisms.
Thus, it is assumed that these methods would act synergistically to overcome
the low permeability of the most apical layer of the skin, the SC, leading to an
enhanced drug penetration. Among physical enhancement methods, especially microneedles (MNs), iontophoresis, ultrasound, and electroporation, are
being used together with nanocarriers to induce a synergistic penetration
enhancement of drugs into/through the skin (Park et al., 2010; Rastogi et al.,
2010; Elsabahy and Foldvari, 2013; Balázs et al., 2016; Charoenputtakun
et al., 2015). Thus, invasomes being potent nanocarriers, have been intensively studied when applied together with different physical methods
(Table 3.2).

3.6.1 Invasomes Combined With Microneedles

Vesicles are often used in combination with microneedles (MNs) with the aim
to further enhance the drug penetration/permeation through the skin. MNs are
micron-sized needles with a height of 10-2000 μm and a width of 10-50 μm,
which can penetrate through the epidermis layer to the dermal tissue directly
without pain (Hao et al., 2017). MNs have been used frequently as they facilitate intra/transdermal delivery of drugs in a minimally invasive fashion (Dul
et al., 2017; Ripolin et al., 2017; Ye et al., 2018; Singh et al., 2019; Jamaledin
et al., 2020). Recently they have been started to be extensively investigated for
their use in dermatology (Sabri et al., 2019). In brief, the mechanism of action
of MNs is based on creating transiently microconduits, which penetrate through
the stratum corneum, extend into the viable epidermis and hence facilitate drug

TABLE 3.2 Invasomes combined with physical enhancement methods for dermal and transdermal drug delivery

FORMULATION	DRUG	INDICATION	CONDITION	OUTCOME	REF.
Invasomes 10% PC, 1% w/v terpene mixture (cineole:citral:d-limonene = 0.45:0.45:0.10 v/v), 3.3 % w/v ethanol and Dermaroller® (needle lenght 150, 500, 1500 μm)	Radiolabeled mannitol	Hydrophilic model drug	In vitro, human skin	Dermaroller® with a needle length of 500 μm showed highest delivery of hydrophilic compound into deeper skin layers or through the skin.	(Badran et al., 2009)
Invasomes Terpenes (limonene, carvone and nerolidol; 0.5, 1, 1.5% w/v) And iontophoresis (0.5 mA/cm2, 3:1 pulse on/off ratio)	Finasteride	Benign prostatic hyperplasia	Ex vivoWistar rat skin	Invasomes containing 0.5% of the lipophilic terpene limonene enhanced the drug flux by 21.17 fold when compared to control aqueous solution, thus, exhibiting highest penetration enhancement of finasteride. Applied together with iontophoresis these invasomes enhanced	(Prasanthi et al., 2013).

(Continued)

TABLE 3.2 (Continued) Invasomes combined with physical enhancement methods for dermal and transdermal drug delivery

FORMULATION	DRUG	INDICATION	CONDITION	OUTCOME	REF.
				drug flux by 25.83 fold when compared to control aqueous solution. Relative bioavailability of 303% was obtained with the invasomal gel comapred to oral drug administration.	
Invasomes (1% v/v, limonene, fenchone and anethole) and iontophoresis	Tolterodine tartrate	Overactive bladder	Ex vivo Wistar rat skin	Invasomes containing 1% limonene provided highest percutaneous penetration being 3.4 fold higher than that of the control. Iontophoresis used together with invasomes, exhibited an additive effect of applied methods on the flux of tolterodine tartrate.	(Kalpana and Lakshmi, 2013)

Formulation	Drug	Indication/Purpose	Model	Result	Reference
Invasomes drug: lipid ratios (1:10 or 1:7.5), 0.75% or 1.5%, w/v terpenes (limonene, cineole, fenchone or citral) and sonophoresis (low frequency, continuous mode for 15 min at a 100% duty cycle)	Agomelatine	Melatonergic antidepressant	Ex vivo, Wistar rat skin/in vivo, rabbits	Invasomes led in rabbits to a significantly higher C_{max} and relative bioavailability ($\approx$ 7.25 folds) compared to agomelatine oral dispersion.	(Tawfik et al., 2020)
Invasomes 10% PC, 1% w/v terpene mixture (cineole:citral:d-limonene = 0.45:0.45:0.10 v/v), 3.3 % w/v ethanol and massage	Fluorescent dyes (CF and DOPE-rhodamine)	Investigating the depth of vesicle penetration	Ex vivo, human skin	Massage increased significantly the follicular penetration of both conventional liposomes and invasomes.	(Trauer et al., 2014)

permeation, as well as the penetration of drug carriers. It represents a powerful enhancement method, when used alone, e.g. for intradermal vaccination and gene delivery (Dul et al., 2017; Sala et al., 2018; Sabri et al., 2020), intradermal delivery of cosmetic actives (Puri et al., 2016), transdermal delivery of insulin and other drugs (Sabri et al., 2020; Kearney et al., 2016), as well as combined with other physical methods, such as with iontophoresis (Ronnander et al., 2019), electroporation (Fang et al., 2001) and sonophoresis (Chen et al., 2009). Also the combination of ultrasonic waves and iontophoresis with MNs has been reported (Bok et al., 2020). For more details on MNs, the reader should refer to (McAlister et al., 2017; Vicente-Perez et al., 2017; Gomaa et al., 2012).

Badran et al. (2009) have shown that invasomes containing besides SPC, 1% w/v of the terpene mixture (cineole:citral:d-limonene = 0,45:0,45:0,10 v/v) and 3.3% w/v ethanol were more effective in delivering hydrophilic radiolabeled mannitol *in vitro* into and through human skin compared to the aqueous drug solutions. The amount of radiolabeled mannitol in the SC and in the stripped skin was 3.8 and 5.7-fold higher for invasomes compared to the buffer solution. The authors additionally applied the microneedle device Dermaroller® in order to induce skin perforation and, hence, further enhancement of drug penetration and permeation into/through the skin

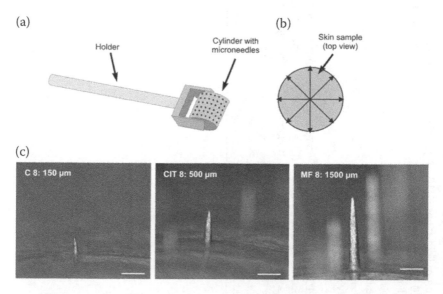

FIGURE 3.11 Schematic presentation of a Dermaroller® (A), of skin perforation (B) and stereo microscopic images (Leica MZ 8,Switzerland) of the needles of the different models of Dermarollers® (C). Bars represent 500 <μm (Badran et al., 2009).

(Figure 3.11). The Dermaroller® with 150 μm long needles used together with invasomes provided the highest drug amount in the SC (1.4-fold higher) and an increased drug amount in the stripped skin (3.1-fold higher) as well as in the receptor fluid (13.6-fold higher) compared to invasomes applied alone. Increasing the needle length from 150 to 500 and 1500 μm, led to an increase of mannitol deposition into deeper skin layers and the receptor fluid, while mannitol amounts in the SC were reduced, i.e. the amounts of mannitol were 8.7- and 6.5-fold higher in the stripped skin (deeper skin) and 30.3- and 49.2-fold higher in the receptor fluid (for 500 and 1500 μm needle lengths, respectively) compared to the application of only invasomes (Figure 3.12). Penetration and fluorescence microscopy studies showed that the Dermaroller® with a needle length of 500 μm provided highest drug deposition in the deeper skin layers (Table 3.2). As to the Dermaroller® with the longest needles of 1500 μm, it may reach deeper regions of the underlying dermis with risk of pain and damage of small blood capillaries. According to the authors, the Dermaroller® with a needle length of 500 μm appeared most promising for the delivery of hydrophilic compounds from invasomes into deeper skin layers or through the skin (Badran et al., 2009).

3.6.2 Invasomes Combined With Ultrasound

Vesicles may be used together with ultrasound. Percutaneous penetration enhancement induced by ultrasound (termed also sonophoresis) indicates that the enhanced transport of molecules is under the influence of ultrasound. Various frequencies of ultrasound (in the range of 20 kHz–16 MHz) have been used to enhance skin permeability. However, transdermal drug delivery induced by low-frequency ultrasound ($f < 100$ kHz) has been found to be more efficient than that induced by high frequency ultrasound. This method has been used to enhance transdermal transport of various drugs including macromolecules (Mitragotri, 2017). For more information on ultrasound, the reader should refer to references (Lee et al., 2017; Mitragotri, 2017).

Tawfik et al. (2020) developed invasomes loaded with agomelatine, the first melatonergic antidepressant. Their aim was to enable its transdermal delivery since the oral drug administration is limited due to low oral bioavailability (<5%) as the drug undergoes extensive hepatic metabolism. Agomelatine-loaded invasomes were developed using two drug: lipid ratios (1:10 or 1:7.5), four different terpenes (limonene, cineole, fenchone or citral), and two terpene concentrations (0.75% or 1.5%, w/v). The effect of the different formulation variables on the characteristics of the developed agomelatine-loaded invasomes was studied by the $2^2.4^1$ full factorial design

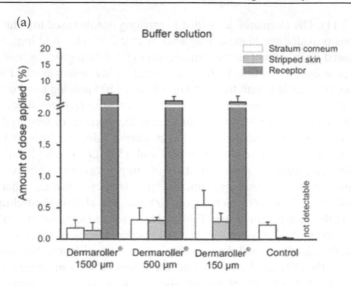

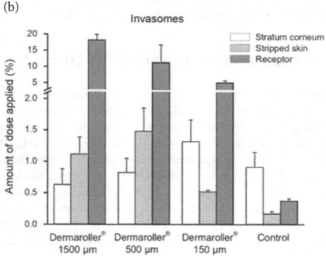

FIGURE 3.12 Amount of radiolabeled mannitol delivered into the SC, stripped skin (deeper skin layers) and the receptor after 6 h of incubation in dependence on the formulation (A) buffer solution and Dermaroller®, (B) invasomes and Dermaroller® treatment (n = 3). The controls present the skin samples without Dermaroller® treatment (Badran et al., 2009).

using Design-Expert® software (Stat-Ease, Inc., Minneapolis, MN). Among different invasomes, three formulations, i.e. invasomes with 0.75% limonene, invasomes with 1.5 % limonene, and invasomes with 1.5% cineole (drug to

PC ratio, 1:10, for all invasomes), were selected for further investigations, such as the *ex vivo* permeation study in newborn Wistar rat skin. Agomelatine-loaded invasomes provided a significantly higher value of the cumulative amount of drug permeated (Q_{24h}) and flux compared to the oral dispersion of the drug. Invasomes containing agomelatine and PC at ratio of 1:10, 1.5 % limonene exhibited the highest permeation enhancing effect, as they provided a Q_{24h} of 214.3 $\mu g/cm^2$ and flux of 10.8 $\mu g/cm^2$ /h compared to Q_{24h} of 53.1 $\mu g/cm^2$ and flux of 2.2 ± 0.1 $\mu g/cm^2$/h obtained by the oral drug dispersion, thus, showing an enhancement ratio of 4.8. The authors attributed this to the synergistic effect of ethanol and terpenes on drug permeation, as it has been shown previously that terpenes together with ethanol lead to an increase of drug flux due to lipid extraction from the SC, macroscopic barrier perturbation, and the enhancement in drug partitioning to the SC (Zhao and Singh, 1999). Similar results were obtained for invasomes loaded with dapsone, temoporfin, and other drugs (Dragicevic-Curic et al., 2008; El-Nabarawi et al., 2018). Further, these invasomes were of small size (313 nm), high zeta potential (-64 mV) and high EE% (78.6%), and also provided high drug released percentages after 0.5h ($Q_{0.5h}$) of 30.1% and after 8 h (Q_{8h}) of 92%. These optimized invasomes were incorporated into the HPMC (0.5% w/v) gel. The obtained agomelatine-loaded invasomal gel was applied together with sonophoresis at optimal conditions, i.e. which involved application of low frequency ultrasound in the continuous mode for 15 min at a 100% duty cycle. Agomelatine-loaded invasomes led in rabbits to a significantly higher C_{max} and relative bioavailability ($\approx$7.25 folds) and a similar T_{max} (0.5 h) compared to agomelatine oral dispersion. According to the authors, significantly improved agomelatine bioavailability could be attributed to several factors including: (1) lipophilic nature of agomelatine (optimum log P value = 2.83), (2) avoidance of the first pass metabolism, (3) high surface area to volume ratio of invasomes which promotes the intimate drug contact with the skin, (4) permeation enhancement effect of invasomes due to the synergistic effects of PC, ethanol and limonene, and (5) the influence of sonophoresis which temporarily increases the skin permeability in a non-invasive manner (Tawfik et al., 2020). Thus, it has been shown that invasomes combined with ultrasound represent a promising transdermal delivery system for agomelatine.

3.6.3 Invasomes Combined With Massage

Trauer et al. (2014) investigated *ex vivo* in human skin the influence of massage and occlusion, on the follicular penetration depth of invasomes and conventional rigid liposomes being loaded with both a hydrophilic dye and a lipophilic dye. 1,2-Dioleoyl-sn-glycero-3-phosphoethanolamine-N-(lissamine rhodamineB), ammonium salt (Rh-DOPE) as a lipophilic fluorescent dye was located in the liposomal membrane, while CF as a hydrophilic fluorescent dye was enclosed into the aqueous core of the liposomes. Conventional liposomes penetrated to a depth of 93.2 μm, while invasomes were seen at the depth of 137.3 μm, when applied without massage, revealing that neither the sebaceous glands nor the bulge region was reached. However, when massage was applied liposomes and invasomes penetrated to a depth of 477.2 μm and 698.8 μm, respectively, which enabled the target sites to be reached (Figure 3.13). Thus, massage, as a physical penetration enhancing method, increased significantly the follicular penetration of both conventional liposomes and invasomes (Table 3.2). Independent of the massage application, the flexible liposomes penetrated significantly deeper than the rigid liposomes. In contrast, occlusion increased follicular penetration depth only of

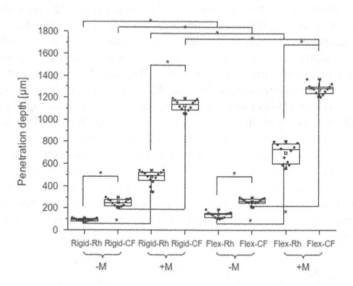

FIGURE 3.13 Massage effect follicular penetration depths of rigid (Rigid) and flexible (Flex) liposomes, i.e. invasomes with (+M) and without (M) massage appliance. Rh-DOPE (Rh) was used as a label for the liposome bilayer and CF for the inner, aqueous liposome core (n = 6; *p < 0.05) (Trauer et al., 2014).

rigid liposomes. The finding that invasomes did not penetrate more effectively when occlusion was applied was expected as for deformable liposomes transepidermal water gradient is needed for an efficient skin penetration (Cevc et al., 1998). The results confirmed that massage is a potent tool for increasing follicular penetration of vesicles.

3.7 *IN VIVO* AND *IN VITRO* THERAPEUTIC EFFECTIVENESS OF INVASOMES

3.7.1 Invasomes in the Treatment of *Alopecia Areata*

The studies on the therapeutic effectiveness of invasomes are listed in Table 3.3. In order to prove the therapeutic effectiveness of CsA-loaded invasomes, Verma *et al.* used 0,5% CsA-loaded invasomes containing 2% w/v standard terpene mixture (cineole:citral:d-limonene = 0.45:0.45:0.10 v/v) and 3.3 % w/v ethanol in the treatment of *Alopecia areata* in the Dundee Experimental Bald Rat (DEBR) model (Verma et al., 2004). CsA-loaded invasomes were compared to conventional liquid-state CsA-loaded liposomes and to the CsA-ethanolic solution. Hence, fifteen rats were divided into three groups. All rats were treated with formulations of CsA twice a day for 6 weeks within a bald flank, while the contralateral flank received an equivalent control formulation. The obtained results suggested that CsA-liposomes with (invasomes) and without terpenes (conventional liposomes) have promising potential as a topical treatment for *Alopecia areata*, showing hair regrowth, reduced inflammatory infiltrate and improved hair follicle morphology on treated sites. Invasomes induced a faster visible hair regrowth on the drug treated site than conventional liposomes (Figure 3.14). In contrast, the ethanolic solution of CsA showed neither visible signs of hair growth nor reduction of hair follicle inflammation. The results indicated that CsA in liposomes provided a localized hair growth promoting effect, while the synergistic effect of ethanol, terpenes, and phospholipids might be an explanation for the enhanced delivery of CsA by invasomes and accumulation of the vesicles in the hair follicles, this, inducing their faster therapeutic effectiveness (Verma et al., 2004).

TABLE 3.3 In vitro and in vivo therapeutic effectiveness of invasomes

FORMULATION	DRUG	INDICATION	CONDITION	OUTCOME	REF.
Invasomes 10% w/v PC, 2% w/v terpene mixture (cineole:citral:d-limonene = 45:45:10 v/v), 3.3 % w/v ethanol	Lipophilic drug Cyclosporine A (CsA)	Alopecia areata	In vivo, DEBR model	Invasomes induced a faster visible hair regrowth on the drug treated site than conventional liposomes.	(Verma et al., 2004)
Invasomes 10% w/v PC, 1% w/v citral, 1% w/v terpene mixture (cineole:citral:d-limonene=45:45:10 v/v), ethanolic drug solution	Hydrophobic drug Temoporfin (mTHPC)	Topical PDT	In vivo, mice	Invasomes containing 1% w/v terpene mixture, being the most efficient formulation induced only a slower tumor growth compared to the control.	(Dragicevic-Curic et al., 2008)
Invasomes 10% w/v PC, 1% w/v citral, 1% w/v terpene mixture (cineole:citral:d-limonene=45:45:10 v/v), ethanolic drug solution	Hydrophobic drug Temoporfin (mTHPC)	Topical PDT	In vitro, A431 and HT29 cells	A431 cells, were more sensitive to PDT with mTHPC-formulations than HT29 cells, and mTHPC-invasomes were more cytotoxic in A431 cells compared to ethanolic drug solution.	(Dragicevic-Curic et al., 2010)
Liposomes, invasomes, DDAB and CTAB LeciPlex	Azelaic acid Idebenone	Anti-acne drug Antioxidant (anticancer) drug	Ex vivo, human skinIn vivo, rats	LeciPlex increased delivery of idebenone whereas invasomes increased delivery of azelaic acid in ex vivo experiments. Azelaic acid invasomal gels showed the highest in vivo anti-acne activity.	(Shah et al., 2015)

Invasomes	Isradipine	Antihypertensive drug	In vivo, Wistar rats	Invasomes induced a 17.43% reduction in blood pressure at a 4h time point and the blood pressure was controlled for up to 24 h.	(Qadri et al., 2017)
Conventional liposomes: cholesterol (0.5% w/v), soya PC (3% w/v); Invasomes: d-limonene (1% w/v), 10% (v/v) ethanol, transfersomes: sodium deoxycholate (15% w/w related to lipid content)	Phenylethyl rezorcinol	Skin lightening agent	In vitro, B16 melanoma cells	Transfersomes and invasomes exerted higher activity in both tyrosinase inhibition and melanin content reduction compared to conventional liposomes.	(Amnuaikit et al., 2018)
Invasomes Fenchone (2.5, 4%) Invasomal gel (4% fenchone)	Anastrozole	Breast cancer	Ex vivo Wistar rat skin	Invasomal gel (4% fenchone) delivered a 13.11-fold higher anastrozole amount into the skin compared to the control gel and showed in MCF-7 cancer cells cytotoxic effect (at 5 µL/mL).	(Vidya and Lakshmi, 2019)
Invasomes containing thymol, menthol, camphor and 1,8-cineol	Terpenes are active ingredients	Antimicrobial agents	In vitro, against S. aureus and E. coli	Thymol containing invasomes showed a strong selective activity against Gram-positive bacteria.	(Kaltschmidt et al., 2020).

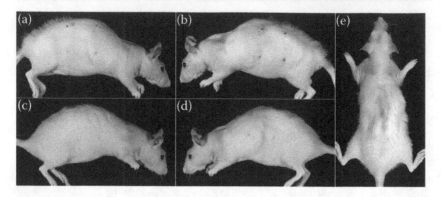

FIGURE 3.14   Hair growth before and after treatment of DEBR with CsA-loaded invasomes. At the start of therapy, complete loss of hair on the flanks can be seen within and beyond the marked area, as well as hair loss on head and shoulders (a, b). After 6 weeks of topical application of CsAloaded invasomes, the treated area is fully rehaired with some hair fibers longer than would be expected with a normal rat pelage (c). Control-treated skin did not show any growth of hair (d) as compared to the drug-treated skin (c, e) (Verma et al., 2004).

3.7.2 Invasomes in Photodynamic Therapy and Anti-Cancer Therapy

Two mTHPC-invasome dispersions, invasomes with 1% w/v citral and invasomes with 1% w/v standard terpene mixture (penetration enhancer (PE) mix), as well as the ethanolic mTHPC solution were used for PDT of mice bearing the subcutaneously (s.c.) implanted human colorectal carcinoma HT29 (Dragicevic-Curic et al., 2008). This pilot PDT study was performed with the aim to test whether the chosen mTHPC-loaded invasomes can reduce tumor size by PDT or at least slow down tumor growth compared to the control group (mice without any treatment). mTHPC-invasomes containing 1% w/v terpene mixture, even exhibiting the highest effectiveness among mTHPC-loaded formulations, were not able to reduce the HT29 tumor size. However, their application induced a slower tumor growth compared to the control, despite the high invasivity, intermediate sensitivity to PDT and subcutaneous localization of the HT29 carcinoma, which limited the success of PDT. Thus, these results, despite not showing a tumor decrease, are promising and indicate that mTHPC-loaded invasomes might be a good modality for the PDT treatment of skin disorders that are more sensitive to PDT, less invasive, and more accessible, like psoriasis or different superficial skin tumors (such as Bowen's disease, basal cell carcinoma).

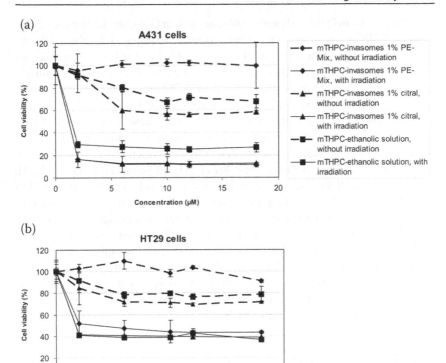

FIGURE 3.15 Dark and photocytotoxicity of three mTHPC-formulations used at different THPC-concentrations against A431 and HT29 tumor cells after 24 h of incubation. For the photocytotoxicity study tumor cells were photoirradiated with a light dose of 20 J/cm². (A) A431 cells and (B) HT29 cells (Dragicevic-Curic et al., 2010).

The aforementioned mTHPC-loaded invasomes containing 1% w/v citral or 1% w/v terpene mixture, and the ethanolic solution of mTHPC, which were used in the PDT of mice bearing the s.c. implanted tumor HT29 (Dragicevic-Curic et al., 2008), were further investigated for their photodynamic efficacy *in vitro* in two tumor cell lines, i.e. in the human epidermoid carcinoma cell line A431 and the human colorectal carcinoma cell line HT29 (Dragicevic-Curic et al., 2010). The results revealed that invasomes and ethanolic solution used at a 2 μM mTHPC-concentration, incubation time 24 h and photo-irradiation at 20 J/cm² were able to reduce survival of HT29 cells and especially of A431 cells, which were more sensitive to PDT (Figure 3.15). In contrast to HT29 cells, where there was not a significant difference between cytotoxicity of mTHPC-ethanolic solution and mTHPC-invasomes, in A431 cells mTHPC-invasomes were more cytotoxic compared to the ethanolic solution. Namely, the incubation of cells with the 2 µM mTHPC-formulations decreased cell viability to 16% and 30% for the mTHPC-invasomes with 1% citral or 1% of the terpene mixture and mTHPC-ethanolic solution, respectively. With the increase of mTHPC-concentration from 2 to 18 µM, cell viability did not show a remarkable continuous decrease. Cell viability ended at 12% and 27% for the 18 µM invasomes with 1% citral or 1% terpene mixture and the ethanolic solution, respectively, which did not significantly differ from the values obtained with lower mTHPC-concentrations of 2 µM. Thus, the low cell survival of about 16% for A431 cells treated with 2 µM of invasome formulations is very promising, since it demonstrates invasomes' high potential to be used in topical PDT of cutaneous malignant diseases.

MCF-7 breast cancer cell line a cytotoxic effect when used at 5 µL/mL at 72 h. Authors have shown that the anastrozole-loaded invasomal gel is able to increase the anastrozole amount in the skin and to exhibit the cytotoxic effect, and, thus, can be used to target drug action in the treatment of breast cancer in postmenopausal women, overcoming the problem of oral administration of anastrozole (Vidya and Lakshmi, 2019).

3.7.3 Invasomes in Treatment of *Acne Vulgaris*

Acne vulgaris is a widespread skin disorder affecting 95% of population. *Azelaic acid* is a derivative of oleic acid with anti-keratinizing and bacteriostatic activities against aerobic and anaerobic bacteria (Sieber and Hegel, 2013). Due to its keratolytic and antibacterial activity, it is efficient for the treatment of *Acne vulgaris*, i.e. it is effective in the treatment of comedones and inflammatory lesions (Waller et al., 2006). To increase its efficacy and decrease its side effects, it has been incorporated in this study into different nanocarriers, i.e. liposomes, invasomes and cationic LeciPlex (Shah et al., 2015). The LeciPlex systems were composed of SPC, a cationic agent, and a biocompatible solvent like polyethylene glycol (PEG) 300, PEG 400, Transcutol® HP (diethylene glycol monoethyl ether), glyco-furol (tetrahydrofurfuryl alcohol polyethylene glycol ether), Soluphor® P (2-pyrrolidone) or Pharmasolve™ (N-methyl-2-pyrrolidone) (Date et al., 2011). As cationic surfactant cetyltrimethylammonium bromide (CTAB) and didodecyldimethyl ammonium bromide (DDAB) were used. These three nanocarriers were loaded with azelaic acid as an antiacne drug, but also with the antioxidant/anticancer drug idebenone used in the management of melanoma (Wempe et al., 2009). As to their particle size and homogeneity, LeciPlex formulations had higher particle size and PDI, i.e., ranging from approximately 260 nm to 350 nm and from 0.2 to 0.4, respectively, as they were prepared using a single step mixing without homogenization. In contrast, invasomes were of small particle size and high homogeneity, as their size was approximately 140 nm with PDI < 0.1. As to liposomes, when loaded with idebenone their size was approximately 288 nm with PDI of 0.4, while azelaic acid-loaded liposomes were smaller, i.e. 147 nm and with a PDI of 0.4. Leciplex carriers possessed a high positive surface charge, while liposomes were neutral and invasomes possessed a slightly negative surface charge. The entrapment efficiency for both idebenone- and azelaic acid-loaded vesicular systems was more than 90%. The ability of these three vesicular systems to enhance the percutaneous penetration of azelaic acid and idebenone was studied *ex vivo* in human skin. The results revealed that LeciPlex carriers provided higher percutaneous penetration for idebenone, i.e. CTAB LeciPlex deposited the highest amount of idebenone, with 0.7% of the total applied drug reaching different layers of the skin. In contrast, invasomes provided higher penetration of azelaic acid as they deposited 5.75% of the total drug amount applied and could be detected in different layers of the skin (Figure 3.16).

The penetration of the lipophilic fluorescent dye (2Z)-2-[(E)-3-(3,3-dimethyl-1-octadecylindol-1-ium-2-yl)prop-2-enylidene]-3,3-dimethyl-1-octadecylindole perchlorate] (DiI) from different carriers was also investigated *ex vivo* in human skin by CLSM in order to clarify the differences in the penetration behavior of the three vesicular systems. The highest fluorescence intensity was observed for the cationic LeciPlex formulations followed by invasomes and liposomes. Invasomes loaded with DiI reached also deep hair follicles, however, in much lower concentration than Leciplex carriers. The authors proposed that LeciPlex carriers employ a dual pathway for skin delivery, the transfollicular and the intercellular pathway compared to the mainly intercellular pathway for invasomes and liposomes (Shah et al., 2015).

As to the therapeutic efficacy in the treatment of acne, invasomal gels obtained by incorporation of azelaic acid-loaded vesicles into a 2% Methocel™K4M gel exhibited the best anti-acne efficacy *in vivo* in rats, followed by liposomal gels and DDAB LeciPlex gels showing similar activity and CTAB LeciPlex gels showing the least activity (Figure 3.17). Invasomal gels showed significantly faster and better activity as compared to other delivery systems from day 2 through day 7, while by day 10, all the delivery systems had achieved similar antiacne activity, but at different rates. All vesicular gels exhibited significantly better *in vivo* activity when compared to azelaic acid suspension. As to the *in vitro* antimicrobial study of azelaic acid loaded in different nanocarriers against *Propionibacterium acne,* it revealed high antimicrobial activity when encapsulated in DDAB LeciPlex followed by almost equal activity for invasomes and CTAB LeciPlex, followed by liposomes. Idebenone loaded nanocarriers were investigated for their cytotoxicity in B16F10 melanoma cell lines and it has been shown that idebenone-loaded LeciPlex formulations were superior followed by invasomes and liposomes (Shah et al., 2015).

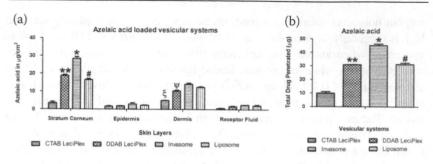

FIGURE 3.16 (A) Ex vivo human skin penetration (mg/cm^2) of vesicular systems loaded with azelaic acid. A significant difference in azelaic acid content in stratum corneum between invasomes (*) and all other vesicular systems was observed as well as in stratum corneum between liposome (#) and CTAB LeciPlex; DDAB LeciPlex (**) and CTAB LeciPlex. In dermis, significant difference between CTAB LeciPlex (j) and liposome, invasomes, and DDAB LeciPlex (C). (B) Total azelaic acid penetration from all layers of the skin. A significant difference between invasomes (*) and other vesicular systems was detected as well as between liposome (#) and CTAB LeciPlex, DDAB LeciPlex (**) and CTAB LeciPlex. Error bars represent SEM (n = 6) (Shah et al., 2015).

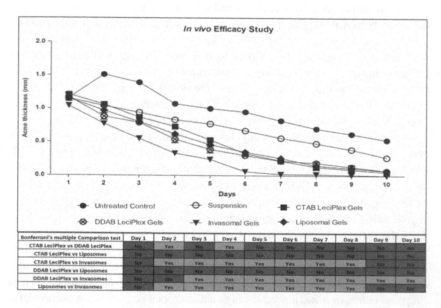

FIGURE 3.17 In vivo anti-acne efficacy study in rats with CTAB LeciPlex, DDAB LeciPlex, invasomes, and liposome loaded with azelaic acid. Bonferroni's multiple comparison test was applied to determine statistical difference between delivery systems on different days, which are tabulated. Error bars represent SEM (n = 6) (Shah et al., 2015).

3.7.4 Invasomes in the Treatment of Hypertension

Isradipine-loaded invasomes were investigated for their therapeutic effectiveness in the treatment of hypertension. Before their application onto the skin, invasomes were incorporated into a 2% carbomer (Carbopol® 934) gel. The antihypertensive study performed *in vivo* in Wistar rats, demonstrated a substantial and constant decrease in blood pressure in the group treated with isradipine-loaded invasomal gel, for up to 24 h. The isradipine-loaded invasomes were highly effective, inducing a 17.43% reduction in blood pressure at a 4h time point. Upon the application of the invasomal gel, the blood pressure of hypertensive rats was controlled for up to 24 h. At 8–24 h time point the applied invasomal gel maintained the blood pressure in the range of normal blood pressure value and the effect was continued till 24 h (Figure 3.18). Thus, the authors developed isradipine invasomes able to enhance the transdermal drug flux and decrease blood pressure in rats, thereby representing a promising formulation for the potential management of hypertension (Qadri et al., 2017).

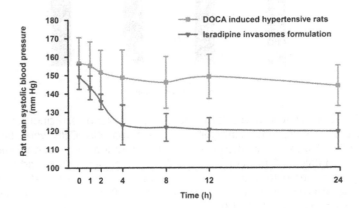

FIGURE 3.18 Blood pressure lowering effect of applied isradipine-loaded invasomal gel in DOCA induced hypertensive rats. Hypertension was induced in two groups of rats by allowing them to drink 1% NaCl in drinking water and by injecting deoxycorticosterone acetate (DOCA, 5 mg/kg in corn oil) subcutaneously at every fourth day for 2 weeks. After 2 weeks, one group was treated with isradipine-loaded invasomal gel (Qadri et al., 2017).

3.7.5 Invasomes for Skin Lightening

In vitro accumulation of *phenylethyl resorcinol* in full-thickness newborn pig skin demonstrated that the application of elastic vesicles, i.e. invasomes and transfersomes, provided significantly higher drug accumulation than liposomes (see Section 3.5.4.) and gave anti-tyrosinase activity up to 80%. Afterwards, these drug-loaded vesicles were tested *in vitro* in B16 melanoma cells for their efficacy in tyrosinase inhibition and melanin content reduction (Figure 3.19). Obtained results showed that transfersomes and invasomes exerted higher activity in both tyrosinase inhibition and melanin content reduction compared to conventional liposomes, being in accordance with skin permeation studies (Amnuaikit et al., 2018).

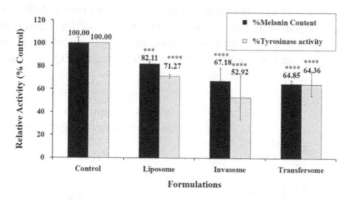

FIGURE 3.19 Effects of vesicles containing phenylethyl rezorcinol on melanin production and tyrosinase activity in B16 melanoma cells. Cells were stimulated with 100 nM α-MSH and then treated with indicating formulations (each formulation containing 5 µM PR) for 72 h. Cellular melanin content and tyrosinase activity were measured and analyzed. Bars represent the means ±S.D. of three independent experiments (n = 3). ****$P < 0.01$, ***$P < 0.05$ compared with the control (Amnuaikit et al., 2018).

3.7.6 Invasomes in Treatment of Bacterial Infections

Invasomes containing thymol, menthol, camphor, and 1,8-cineol, were prepared, characterized, and investigated for their bactericidal properties against *S. aureus* and *E. coli*, as terpenoids have besides strong antioxidant and anti-inflammatory effects also antimicrobial properties (Kaltschmidt et al., 2020).

Terpenes are mostly used as permeation enhancers to enhance dermal and transdermal drug delivery rather than being bioactive components. However, in this study authors investigated invasomes encapsulating these terpenes as bioactive components for their efficacy to inhibit bacterial cell growth. The results revealed that thymol-containing invasomes led to the strongest growth inhibition of *S. aureus*, while camphor- or cineol-containing invasomes mediated cell death, whereas menthol-containing invasomes did not affect the growth of *S. aureus*. Flow cytometric analysis confirmed that thymol-containing invasomes were highly bactericidal to *S. aureus*. In contrast, thymol-containing invasomes did not affect the survival of Gram-negative *E. coli*. Cineole-containing invasomes induced a strong growth inhibition of *E.coli*. The authors concluded that particularly thymol-containing invasomes showed a strong selective activity against Gram-positive bacteria and, thus, they could be used for the treatment of severe bacterial infections (e.g. caused by methicillin-resistant *S. aureus*) in nose, lung and skin wounds (Kaltschmidt et al., 2020).

3.8 FLUIDITY OF INVASOMES

Penetration studies investigating different invasomes described in previous sections have shown that invasomes dependent on the added terpene or terpene mixture may represent vesicles with a high penetration enhancing ability. The physicochemical properties of liposomes can affect the skin penetration of their entrapped drugs (Van Kuijk-Meuwissen et al., 1998; Verma et al., 2003; Van Kuijk-Meuwissen et al., 1998; Song and Kim, 2006). Among all properties, the fluidity, i.e. the thermodynamic state of their bilayers, influences at most the penetration enhancing ability of liposomes. As liquid-state (fluid) vesicles have been found to be superior over gel state (rigid) vesicles in terms of increasing the drug penetration into the skin (Van Kuijk-Meuwissen et al., 1998; El Maghraby et al., 1999; El Maghraby et al., 2001; Van Kuijk-Meuwissen et al., 1998), it was assumed that invasomes, showing high penetration enhancing ability (Dragicevic-Curic et al., 2008; Dragicevic-Curic et al., 2009), would possess high membrane fluidity.

In order to confirm this assumption, the fluidity of different invasomes was investigated by two methods, ESR and DSC (Dragicevic-Curic et al., 2011). Two spin labels, i.e. 5- and 16-doxyl stearic acid (5- and 16-DSA), oriented with their longest axis parallel to the phospholipids' acyl chains, were used in order to determine the local motional profiles in the two main regions of the lipid bilayer. The radical in the position 5 of the acyl chain (5-

DSA) can determine motional profiles near the polar head group, while the radical in the position 16 of the acyl chain (16-DSA) determines motional profiles at the end of the hydrophobic chain.

The results obtained by ESR measurements revealed that the addition of 1 % w/v of a single terpene or terpene mixture to liposomes containing 3.3% w/v ethanol in order to obtain invasomes increased significantly the phospholipid fluidity near to the C16 atom of their acyl chains, compared to liposomes without terpenes (conventional liposomes and liposomes containing 3.3% w/v ethanol) (Dragicevic-Curic et al., 2011). Thus, ESR showed that invasomes indeed represent vesicles of higher membrane fluidity than conventional liposomes. However, the membrane fluidity did not differ markedly among different invasomes. It was not possible to differentiate between the influences of each single terpene/terpene mixture on the invasome fluidity, and hence there was also no direct correlation between the invasome fluidity and their penetration enhancing ability (Dragicevic-Curic et al., 2008; Dragicevic-Curic et al., 2009). However, conventional liposomes (being in fluid thermodynamic state, but significantly lower than invasomes) provided the second lowest mTHPC-amount in the skin compared to different invasomes (after invasomes with the terpene mixture containing the highest amount of D-limonene). According to ESR data, the addition of all terpenes/terpene mixtures increased the vesicle fluidity, while not all terpenes/terpene mixtures increased the penetration enhancing ability of invasomes to improve the skin delivery of mTHPC compared to conventional liposomes or liposomes containing 3.3 % ethanol ability (Dragicevic-Curic et al., 2009). The ESR results are in agreement with DSC results, which also showed that the addition of 1 % w/v terpenes/terpene mixtures increased the molecular motional freedom of phospholipid acyl chains in invasome bilayers (Dragicevic-Curic et al., 2011). The ESR and DSC results are also in agreement with cryo-electron microscopy investigation (Dragicevic-Curic et al., 2008), which showed that the addition of terpenes had an influence on the shape of vesicles, i.e. besides' spherical vesicles, deformed vesicles of different shapes were also present in invasome dispersions, and an increase of the terpenes' amount resulted in their increased number (Figures 3.3. and 3.4). It was assumed that the addition of terpenes, especially 1% w/v terpenes, to already liquid-state (fluid) liposomes with 3.3% w/v ethanol increased further their membrane fluidity. The obtained invasomes were, thus, of very high membrane fluidity compared to liposomes without terpenes, which was confirmed by cryo-electron microscopy, ESR and DSC measurements.

Since results of ESR, DSC and permeation studies did not show a direct correlation between the fluidity and penetration enhancing ability of invasomes, it was proposed that besides fluidity other phenomena might also be involved in the mechanism of the skin penetration enhancement induced by invasomes.

Hofland et al. (1994) proposed for example two mechanisms for nonionic vesicles to play an important role in the vesicle-skin interactions, leading to an enhanced drug penetration: the penetration enhancing effect of the surfactant molecules and the effect of the vesicular structure. Therefore, in the case of invasomes, besides the effect of the fluid vesicular structure, also the penetration enhancing effect of invasome constituents can be assumed. The constituents of invasomes, i.e. phospholipids, ethanol and terpenes represent potent penetration enhancers (Yokomizo and Sagitani, 1996a,b; El-Kattan et al., 2001), which released from fragmented invasomes could synergistically fluidize the intercellular lipid layers in the SC, and thereby increase the skin penetration of drugs and possibly of small invasomes. However, this is only an assumption. The mechanism by which invasomes induce drug penetration enhancement should be investigated in further experiments.

Since elasticity/deformability is an important feature of deformable vesicles which differentiates them from conventional liposomes, the elasticity of invasomes containing 1% of different single terpenes (1% cineole or citral or limonene) or different concentrations of the standard terpene mixture (1% or 1.5%), as well as of transfersomes and conventional liposomes was investigated (Ntimenou et al., 2012). The authors found by size measurements of deformable vesicles, performed before and after their extrusion through polycarbonate filters, that the particle size of most vesicles did not change significantly after extrusion compared to their original size, except in the case of invasomes containing 1.5% of the terpene mixture. Among all vesicles invasomes containing 1% PE (standard terpene mixture) and invasomes containing 1% limonene-possessed highest fluidity and, thus, elasticity. Most invasomes exhibited higher elasticity than the corresponding control formulation (without terpenes) with the exceptions of invasomes containing 1% citral or 1% cineol, which possessed lower elasticity than control vesicles. The finding that the elasticity of invasomes with 1% limonene and invasomes with 1% of the standard terpene mixture did not differ significantly, indicates that limonene is the most important component in the terpene mixture in terms of increasing vesicles' elasticity. Dwivedi et al. (2017) demonstrated that high concentration of eugenol and lecithin in invasomes induced high deformability of isotretinoin-loaded invasomes. It has been also shown that phenylethyl resorcinol-loaded invasomes possessed a higher degree of deformability (25.26%) than transfersomes (6.63%), while conventional liposomes as rigid vesicles did not show any deformability, as measured after their extrusion through a 200 nm polycarbonate filter, which significantly affected the skin permeation of the drug (Amnuaikit et al., 2018).

3.9 MODE OF ACTION OF INVASOMES

Dragicevic et al. (2016) based on the results of different studies investigating the penetration enhancing ability of invasomes (Verma, 2002; Verma et al., 2004; Dragicevic-Curic et al., 2008; Dragicevic-Curic et al., 2008; Dragicevic-Curic et al., 2009) assumed that the reason for the superior behavior of certain invasomes compared to conventional liposomes, liposomes containing small amounts of ethanol and ethanolic solution, was the presence of terpenes and ethanol in liposomes, i.e. the synergistic effect of ethanol, terpenes and liposomes. Liposomes have been used for years to enhance the skin delivery of various drugs (El Maghraby and Williams, 2009). Further, all constituents of invasomes, i.e. terpenes (El-Kattan et al., 2001; Kunta et al., 1997), as well as ethanol (Berner et al., 1989; Mutalik et al., 2009; Jaimes-Lizcano et al., 2011) and phospholipids (Yokomizo and Sagitani, 1996a,bYokomizo 1996) have also been shown to be very potent penetration enhancers. As to phospholipids, invasomes were made of soya PC, which due to its head group, having a strong enhancing effect, presents a strong penetration promoter (Yokomizo and Sagitani, 1996b). The acyl chains of the PC were unsaturated, which further increased the phospholipids' penetration-enhancing ability (Yokomizo and Sagitani, 1996b). In addition, most studies with invasomes used for PC a commercial phospholipid mixture NAT 8539 (Lipoid AG, Germany) which contained besides PC, also lysophosphatidylcholine, imparting flexibility to the vesicle bilayer and acting as a penetration enhancer. Moreover, synergistic effects of ethanol and terpenes (Vaddi et al., 2002; Ota et al., 2003; Puglia et al., 2001), ethanol and liposomes (Verma and Fahr, 2004; Kirjavainen et al., 1999; Touitou et al., 2000) and ethanol, terpenes and liposomes (Verma, 2002) in enhancing the drug permeation have been reported in the literature.

The following mechanism of the penetration enhancing ability of invasomes was proposed (Dragicevic et al., 2016) due to the results of the group of Prof. A. Fahr (Dragicevic-Curic et al., 2008, 2009; Verma, 2002; Verma and Fahr, 2004; Verma et al., 2004; Dragicevic-Curic et al., 2008), as well as studies performed by other research groups (Cevc and Blume, 1992; Cevc et al., 2002; Honeywell-Nguyen et al., 2002). As invasomes were in all studies applied in finite doses under non-occlusion, a number of concomitant processes could take place (Figure 3.20). Small amounts of ethanol from the invasome dispersion (being outside the vesicles) could be able to fluidize the intercellular SC lipids (Barry, 2001). Further, a high part of invasomes is probably fragmented in their attempt to penetrate into the upper SC layers, which leads to the release of terpenes, ethanol and unsaturated phospholipids.

This would be in agreement with findings of most authors (Hofland et al., 1994; Zellmer et al., 1995; Kirjavainen et al., 1996; Kirjavainen et al., 1999), who propose that vesicles disintegrate at the skin surface and vesicle components (i.e. phospholipids) penetrate molecularly dispersed into the intercellular lipid matrix, where they mix with the intercellular lipids of the SC thereby modifying the lipid layers and leading to enhanced drug penetration. Thus, the released ethanol, terpenes, and unsaturated phospholipids would be free to exert their penetration enhancing effect. It is proposed that these penetration enhancers would synergistically act on fluidizing the intercellular SC lipids, since all of them act via this mechanism (Yokomizo and Sagitani, 1996b; Kirjavainen, Urtti, et al., 1999; Dragicevic-Curic et al., 2011; Chen et al., 2016). This could lead to the formation of microcavities and to an increase of the free volume for drug diffusion (Barry, 2001), which could further increase the diffusion coefficient of the drugs released from vesicles. In addition, also the partitioning of the drug into the intercellular lipid bilayers of the SC would be increased by phospholipids (Kirjavainen et al., 1999), ethanol (Megrab et al., 1995) and terpenes (Williams and Barry, 1991b). However, since the constituents of invasomes, being potent penetration enhancers, act also via other mechanisms, these mechanisms could also have an influence on the enhanced penetration of the drug.

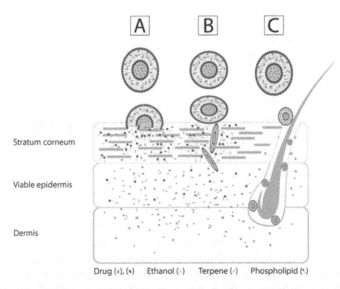

Stratum corneum

Viable epidermis

Dermis

Drug (•), (•)   Ethanol (·)   Terpene (/)   Phospholipid (·)

FIGURE 3.20 Schematic presentation of the penetration enhancing mechanism of invasomes. (A) Penetration enhancement of the free drug induced by phospholipids, terpenes and ethanol, being released due to the desintegration of invasomes, (B) penetration of intact invasomes, (C) transappendageal delivery of invasomes. Completely redrawn and modified from Nangare and Dugam (2020).

Regarding the penetration of vesicles, a lot of phenomena are included which synergistically might facilitate the penetration of some small intact invasomes into the SC, such as: (1) disturbed organization of the SC lipids, (2) high fluidity of invasomes due to the effect of terpenes and ethanol, as confirmed by (Dragicevic-Curic et al., 2011), (3) probably high deformability of invasomes (assumed due to the correlation between vesicles' high fluidity and deformability (Godin and Touitou, 2003), (4) small particle size of vesicles and (5) presence of the transepidermal osmotic gradient, which is an important driving force for the diffusion of intact deformable vesicles of high hydrophilicity as they tend to follow the hydration gradient across the skin (Cevc and Blume, 1992). The release of the drug in the skin layers could be a result of fusion of penetrated vesicles with the intercellular lipids of the SC (Touitou et al., 2000). Verma (2002) proposed a penetration of small invasomes through SC bilayers, disturbed due to the effect of ethanol and terpenes on the SC. Further, according to Verma the pilosebaceous units appeared to be a major route of invasomes' penetration into the skin (Verma, 2002). The penetration of intact deformable vesicles through the skin was proposed by the group of Cevc (Cevc et al., 2002; Cevc and Gebauer, 2003). Honeywell-Nguyen et al. (2002) proposed also a penetration of intact elastic vesicles through channel like regions into the deeper layers of the SC. Touitou et al. (2000) assumed that ethosomes could penetrate into the SC bilayers, being disturbed due to the effect of ethanol. However, penetration of intact vesicles is rejected by most authors (Hofland et al., 1994; Kirjavainen et al., 1999; Zellmer et al., 1995; Kirjavainen et al., 1996).

3.10 THE SAFETY PROFILE OF INVASOMES

Amnuaikit et al. (2018) performed an acute irritation test in rabbits, which was based on erythema and edema formation in 72 h, after the application resorcinol loaded in liposomes, invasomes and transfersomes. The authors confirmed the safety of these formulations for skin application. In contrast to transfersomes which induced slight erythema at 1 h, being recovered after 24 h, the skin area which was treated with the liposomes and invasomes showed no significant differences from the skin area treated with distilled water (controlled area). Thus, the authors confirmed the safety of all vesicles, especially invasomes and liposomes loaded with rezorcinol, for topical application to the skin. Vardenafil hydrochloride-loaded invasomes showed minor histopathologic changes following a leave-on period of 12 h in rats, confirming the safety of invasomes application onto the skin (Ammar et al., 2020). Dragicevic-Curic et al. investigated *in vitro* in A431 and H29 tumor cell lines the cytotoxicity of mTHPC-loaded invasomes after the cells were photoirradiated. However, the authors tested also the dark and light-induced (light dose 20 J/cm^2) cytotoxicity of unloaded invasomes containing 1% citral or invasomes containing 1% of the standard terpene mixture against A431 and HT29 cell lines (24 h incubation with invasomes). The invasomes showed no toxicity against A431 and HT29 cells, since cell viability was always above 86%, indicating the safety of the tested invasomal composition (Figure 3.21). An anastrozole-loaded invasomal gel was tested for its skin irritation in depilated rabbit skin. The reactions at the site of application were assessed and scored according to the Draize method. No erythema and edema were observed even after 72 h, indicating its safety (Vidya and Lakshmi, 2019).

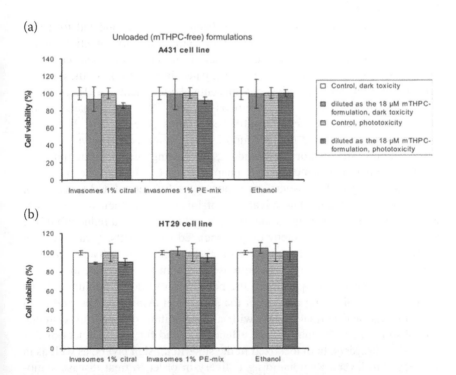

FIGURE 3.21 Dark and photocytotoxicity of unloaded formulations (without mTHPC), i.e. invasomes with 1% terpene mixture (PE), invasomes with 1% citral and ethanolic solution, against tumor cells after 24 h of incubation. For the photocytotoxicity assay, the cells were photoirradiated with a light dose of 20 J/cm^2. (A) A431 cells and (B) HT29 cells (Dragicevic-Curic et al., 2010).

3.11 CONCLUSION

The main problem in dermatopharmacotherapy, i.e. dermal drug delivery, is insufficient drug penetration into the skin, limiting the therapeutic effectiveness of the therapy. As to transdermal drug delivery, the crucial prerequisite is that the drug must be able to permeate through the skin at a sufficiently high rate to achieve therapeutic plasma concentrations. Thus, regardless whether dermal or transdermal drug delivery should be achieved, drug penetration into/through the skin is pivotal, and strategies to overcome the impermeability of the stratum corneum are necessary. In order to circumvent this problem, different penetration enhancement strategies have been used, especially the use of various types of elastic vesicles being nanocarriers for dermal/transdermal drug delivery.

The advantages of invasomes have been recognized and led to a significant development of these nanocarriers attracting the attention of researchers working in the field of dermal and transdermal drug carriers. As a consequence, invasomes have been investigated in numerous studies as carriers for different drugs (active pharmaceutical ingredients, API), cosmetic active ingredients (CAS), and phytoconstituents. Thus, this chapter summarized and discussed recently published studies investigating the use of invasomes as carriers for immunosuppressive, anticancer, antihypertensive, anti-acne, anti-inflammatory, antioxidant, anti-ageing agents, curcumin, etc.

The studies represented in this chapter have highlighted the most important advantages of invasomes as nanocarriers for dermal and transdermal drug delivery. The important advantage of invasomes is their ability to enhance the percutaneous penetration of drugs, which enables a reduction of the drug doses required and thereby drug-associated side effects. Invasomes can be used for targeted drug delivery, i.e. for site-specific drug delivery. Namely, invasomes as a topical drug carrier are used for skin targeting (localized drug effect in the skin), as they enhance the penetration of drugs into/through the SC and increase the drug amount in the superficial skin layers, as well as in the epidermal and dermal layers, with a concomitant decrease of systemic drug absorption. Thus, they can be effectively used for the treatment of different skin disorders, both localized in the superficial skin layers, as well as in the deep skin layers. Regional drug delivery in order to treat disease symptoms in deep tissues beneath the skin surface (e.g. musculature) is also achievable. Due to their particulate structure, they can be used to target the pilosebaceous unit, being promising for the treatment of hair follicle-associated skin disorders, such as acne, alopecia, some skin cancers, etc. (see chapter 2). Invasomes, may also be used for the transdermal drug delivery of drugs, thereby exerting all benefits of transdermal drug delivery, such as avoiding the systemic side effects related to the oral and intravenous drug administration avoiding the gastrointestinal tract, increasing relative bioavailability of the drug by avoiding hepatic first pass, enabling constant plasma levels (controlled drug release, decrease of the pulsed plasma peak level), etc. In order to achieve desired therapeutic effects by invasomes, their penetration enhancing ability should be tailored, by using certain types and concentrations of terpenes and phospholipids. It has been shown, e.g. that the increase of terpene concentration in invasomes increased their penetration enhancing ability up to a concentration of 1.5%, but, decreased invasomes stability above concentrations of 1%. Thus, the concentration of terpenes was mostly adjusted to 1%. It has also been shown that some terpenes/terpene mixtures retarded the drug penetration into the skin compared to liposomes without terpenes, which could be used for targeting the superficial skin layers.

Another benefit of invasomes is their ability to encapsulate both hydrophilic and lipophilic agents. Further, invasomes have been widely used in delivering synthetic drugs as well as drugs from natural sources. It is worth mentioning that invasomes represent a non-invasive penetration enhancement method and that they can be self-administered, which due to these as well as aforementioned benefits increases patient compliance. Furthermore, invasomes are biodegradable, non-toxic, with low allergenic potential, which is advantageous when used in skin diseases, where the SC is already disordered and possesses decreased barrier properties. In addition, the most investigated invasomes contain soy PC, which besides its penetration enhancing ability, is rich in essential fatty acids linoleic and linolenic acid, having a critical role in the skin barrier function (Rhodes, 2000). Linoleic acid has also been shown to be beneficial in the treatment of acne and even psoriasis (which are common therapeutic indications for invasomes), since it restores the skin barrier function and reduces the scaling and epidermal hyperproliferation (Rhodes, 2000; Fluhr and Berardesca, 2000).

The aforementioned properties of invasomes represent important advantages over other passive or active/physical enhancement methods, as they are often used in diseased skin where the use of aggressive formulations/ approaches could further worsen the condition of the diseased skin. However, if required, in order to further enhance percutaneous drug penetration, invasomes may be used in combination with physical enhancement methods. An advantage of invasomes is also their simple preparation, as well as simple application to the skin in contrast to electrically assisted methods, such as iontophoresis, electroporation, sonophoresis, etc.

However, there are also some drawbacks related to the use of invasomes, such as the high cost of invasomes. Stability issues may be also one of the reasons why invasomes did not enter the market. The shelf life of invasomes may be limited due to their potential physical (aggregation/fusion of vesicles) or chemical instability (oxidation/hydrolysis of phospholipids). However, invasomes have been shown to be physically and chemically stable when stored at 4 °C. Further, the scalability (scale-up from laboratory to industry) and reproducibility of invasomes is an important concern for its commercialization. In addition, there is no regulatory guidance on manufacturing requirements to assure the quality of invasomal products. Safety trials regarding acute and chronic toxicity on the use of invasomes are missing, i.e. there are no preclinical and clinical trials on invasomes. All these issues must be addressed before the commercialization of invasomes.

As to the drawbacks of performed research studies, the main problem is that most penetration studies were performed *in vivo* and *in vitro* in healthy skin, which cannot predict precisely a drugs' behavior in disordered skin *in vivo* (if invasomes are intended to be used in the management of skin diseases). Therefore, instead of healthy skin, in future studies skin models should be used which mimic skin diseases, being potential indications for drug-loaded invasomes. Further, studies on invasomes' therapeutic effectiveness *in vitro* and especially *in vivo* are less often performed, despite being of crucial importance. Therefore, researchers should be encouraged to conduct these studies in relevant models. Namely, *in vivo* studies in animal models are needed in order to obtain enough evidence for the potential clinical use of drugs encapsulated in invasomes.

To summarize, the aforementioned invasomes' advantages are very encouraging and invasomes are supposed to enjoy in the near future a period of intense investigation as drug carriers. These positive findings will hopefully lead in the future to the development of commercial invasomal formulations for the treatment of skin disorders, as well as systemic diseases. However, in order to achieve this, future studies must be undertaken to fill in the gaps in the knowledge about invasomes. In addition, besides' described terpenes and terpene mixtures other terpenes and terpene mixtures should be investigated in order to further optimize invasomes' composition, which could lead to the development of invasomes being even more efficient dermal and transdermal drug delivery systems than existing invasomes.

REFERENCES

Abd, E., Benson, H.A.E., Mohammed, Y.H., Roberts, M.S., Grice, J.E., 2019 May 1. Permeation mechanism of caffeine and naproxen through in vitro human epidermis: effect of vehicles and penetration enhancers. *Skin Pharmacol. Physiol.* 32(3), 132–141.

Abdulbaqi, I.M., Darwis, Y., Khan, N.A.K., Assi, R.A., Khan, A.A.. 2016 Ethosomal nanocarriers: the impact of constituents and formulation techniques on ethosomal properties, in vivo studies, and clinical trials. *Int. J. Nanomed.* 11, 2279–2304.

Ahad, A., Aqil, M., Ali, A., 2016 Jun 2. The application of anethole, menthone, and eugenol in transdermal penetration of valsartan: enhancement and mechanistic investigation. *Pharm. Biol.* 54(6), 1042–1051.

Ahad, A., Al-Jenoobi, F.I., Al-Mohizea, A.M., Aqil, M., Kohli, K., 2013. Transdermal delivery of calcium channel blockers for hypertension. *Expert Opin. Drug Deliv.* 10, 1137–1153.

Ahad, A., Al-Saleh, A.A., Akhtar, N., Al-Mohizea, A.M., Al-Jenoobi, F.I., 2015. Transdermal delivery of antidiabetic drugs: formulation and delivery strategies. Vol. 20, *Drug Discovery Today*. Elsevier Ltd. p. 1217–1227.

Ahad, A., Aqil, M., Kohli, K., Chaudhary, H., Sultana, Y., Mujeeb, M., et al., 2009. Chemical penetration enhancers: a patent review. *Expert Opin. Ther. Pat.* 19(7), 969–988.

Ahad, A., Aqil, M., Kohli, K., Sultana, Y., Mujeeb, M., Ali, A., 2011 May. Role of novel terpenes in transcutaneous permeation of valsartan: effectiveness and mechanism of action. *Drug Dev. Ind. Pharm.* 37(5), 583–596.

Ahad, A., Aqil, M., Kohli, K., Sultana, Y., Mujeeb, M., Ali, A., 2011 Feb 7. Interactions between novel terpenes and main components of rat and human skin: mechanistic view for transdermal delivery of propranolol hydrochloride. *Curr. Drug Deliv.* 8(2), 213–224.

Ahad, A., Aqil, M., Kohli, K., Chaudhary, H., Sultana, Y., Mujeeb, M. & Talegaonkar, S., 2009. Chemical penetration enhancers: a patent review. *Expert Opin. Ther. Patents* 19, 969–988.

Ahmed, T.A., 2015 Mar 1. Preparation of transfersomes encapsulating sildenafil aimed for transdermal drug delivery: plackett-Burman design and characterization. *J. Liposome Res.* 25(1), 1–10.

Ahmed, O.A.A., Rizq, W.Y., 2018. Finasteride nano-transferosomal gel formula for management of androgenetic alopecia: ex vivo investigational approach. *Drug Des. Devel. Ther.* 12, 2259–2265.

Ahmed, O.A.A., Badr-Eldin, S.M., 2019 Oct 30. Development of an optimized avanafil-loaded invasomal transdermal film: ex vivo skin permeation and in vivo evaluation. *Int. J. Pharm.* 570, 118657.

Ainbinder, D., Touitou, E., 2005. Testosterone ethosomes for enhanced transdermal delivery. *Drug Deliv. J. Deliv. Target Ther. Agents.* 12(5), 297–303.

Ainbinder, D., Godin, B., Touitou, E. 2016 Ethosomes: Enhanced delivery of drugs to and across the skin. In: *Percutaneous Penetration Enhancers Chemical Methods in Penetration Enhancement*. Nanocarriers.

Ainbinder, D., Paolino, D., Fresta, M., Touitou, E., 2010. Drug delivery applications with ethosomes. *J. Biomed. Nanotechnol.* 6, 558–568.

Al Shuwaili, A.H., Rasool, B.K.A., Abdulrasool, A.A., 2016 May 1. Optimization of elastic transfersomes formulations for transdermal delivery of pentoxifylline. *Eur. J. Pharm. Biopharm.* 102, 101–114.

Ammar, H.O., Tadros, M.I., Salama, N.M., Ghoneim, A.M., 2020. Ethosome-derived invasomes as a potential transdermal delivery system for vardenafil hydrochloride: development, optimization and application of physiologically based pharmacokinetic modeling in adults and geriatrics. *Int. J. Nanomed.* 15, 5671–5685.

Amnuaikit, T., Limsuwan, T., Khongkow, P., Boonme, P., 2018. Vesicular carriers containing phenylethyl resorcinol for topical delivery system; liposomes, transfersomes and invasomes-NC-ND license. *Asian J. Pharm. Sci.* 13, 472–484. http://creativecommons.org/licenses/by-nc-nd/4.0/

Amnuaikit, T., Limsuwan, T., Khongkow, P., Boonme, P., 2018. Vesicular carriers containing phenylethyl resorcinol for topical delivery system; liposomes, transfersomes and invasomes. *Asian J. Pharm. Sci.* 13(5), 472–484.

Aqil, M., Ahad, A., Sultana, Y., Ali, A., 2007. Status of terpenes as skin penetration enhancers. *Drug Discov. Today.* 12(23–24), 1061–1067.

Arya, J., Henry, S., Kalluri, H., McAllister, D.V., Pewin, W.P., Prausnitz, M.R., 2017 Jun 1. Tolerability, usability and acceptability of dissolving microneedle patch administration in human subjects. *Biomaterials* 128, 1–7.

Ascenso, A., Raposo, S., Batista, C., Cardoso, P., Mendes, T., Praça, F.G., et al., 2015 Sep 18. Development, characterization, and skin delivery studies of related ultradeformable vesicles: transfersomes, ethosomes, and transethosomes. *Int. J. Nanomed.* 10, 5837–5851.

Avadhani, K.S., Manikkath, J., Tiwari, M., Chandrasekhar, M., Godavarthi, A., Vidya, S.M., et al., 2017 Feb 3. Skin delivery of epigallocatechin-3-gallate (EGCG) and hyaluronic acid loaded nano-transfersomes for antioxidant and anti-aging effects in UV radiation induced skin damage. *Drug Deliv.* 24(1), 61–74.

Babu, R.J., Pandit, J.K., 2005. Effect of penetration enhancers on the transdermal delivery of bupranolol through rat skin. *Drug Deliv. J. Deliv. Target Ther. Agents.* 12(3), 165–169.

Badran, M.M., Kuntsche, J., Fahr, A., 2009. Skin penetration enhancement by a microneedle device (Dermaroller®) in vitro: dependency on needle size and applied formulation. *Eur. J. Pharm. Sci.* 36(4–5), 511–523.

Badran, M., Shazly, G., El-Badry, M., 2012. Effect of terpene liposomes on the transdermal delivery of hydrophobic model drug, nimesulide: characterization, stability and in vitro skin permeation. *African J. Pharm. Pharmacol.* 6(43), 3018–3026.

Baek, S.H., Shin, J.H., Kim, Y.C., 2017 Mar 1. Drug-coated microneedles for rapid and painless local anesthesia. *Biomed. Microdevices.* 19(1).

Balázs, B., Sipos, P., Danciu, C., Avram, S., Soica, C., Dehelean, C., et al., 2016 Jan 1. ATR-FTIR and Raman spectroscopic investigation of the electroporation-mediated transdermal delivery of a nanocarrier system containing an antitumour drug. *Biomed. Opt. Express.* 7(1), 67.

Barry, B.W., 2001. Novel mechanisms and devices to enable successful transdermal drug delivery. *Eur. J. Pharm. Sci.* 14(2), 101–114.

Benson, H.A.E., 2017. Elastic Liposomes for Topical and Transdermal Drug Delivery. In: *Methods in Molecular Biology.* Humana Press Inc, pp. 107–117.

Berner, B., Mazzenga, G.C., Otte, J.H., Steffens, R.J., Juang, R.H., Ebert, C.D., 1989. Ethanol: water mutually enhanced transdermal therapeutic system II: skin permeation of ethanol and nitroglycerin. *J. Pharm. Sci.* 78(5), 402–407.

Bok, M., Zhao, Z.J., Jeon, S., Jeong, J.H., Lim, E., 2020 Dec 1. Ultrasonically and iontophoretically enhanced drug-delivery system based on dissolving microneedle patches. *Sci. Rep.* 10(1).

Brain, K.R., Green, D.M., Dykes, P.J., Marks, R., Bola, T.S., 2005. The role of menthol in skin penetration from topical formulations of ibuprofen 5% in vivo. *Skin Pharmacol. Physiol.* 19(1), 17–21.

Cevc, G., Blume, G., 1992 Feb 17. Lipid vesicles penetrate into intact skin owing to the transdermal osmotic gradients and hydration force. *BBA - Biomembr.* 1104(1), 226–232.

Cevc, G., Gebauer, D., 2003. Hydration-driven transport of deformable lipid vesicles through fine pores and the skin barrier. *Biophys. J.* 84(2 I), 1010–1024.

Cevc, G., Chopra, A., 2016. Deformable (Transfersome®) vesicles for improved drug delivery into and through the skin. In: *Percutaneous Penetration Enhancers Chemical Methods in Penetration Enhancement: Nanocarriers*. Springer Berlin Heidelberg. 39–59.

Cevc, G., Schätzlein, A., Richardsen, H., 2002. Ultradeformable lipid vesicles can penetrate the skin and other semi-permeable barriers unfragmented. Evidence from double label CLSM experiments and direct size measurements. *Biochim. Biophys. Acta – Biomembr.* 1564(1), 21–30.

Cevc, G., Gebauer, D., Stieber, J., Schätzlein, A., Blume, G., 1998. Ultraflexible vesicles, transfersomes, have an extremely low pore penetration resistance and transport therapeutic amounts of insulin across the intact mammalian skin. *Biochim. Biophys. Acta – Biomembr.* 1368(2), 201–215.

Chang, T.S., 2009. *An updated review of tyrosinase inhibitors.* Vol. 10, International Journal of Molecular Sciences. Molecular Diversity Preservation International. pp. 2440–2475.

Chantasart, D., Pongjanyakul, T., Higuchi, W.I., Li, S.K., 2009. Effects of oxygen-containing terpenes as skin permeation enhancers on the lipoidal pathways of human epidermal membrane. *J. Pharm. Sci.* 98(10), 3617–3632.

Charoenputtakun, P., Li, S.K., Ngawhirunpat, T., 2015. Iontophoretic delivery of lipophilic and hydrophilic drugs from lipid nanoparticles across human skin. *Int. J. Pharm.* 495(1), 318–328.

Chen, M., Liu, X., Fahr, A., 2010. Skin delivery of ferulic acid from different vesicular systems. *J. Biomed. Nanotechnol.* 6(5), 577–585.

Chen, M., Liu, X., Fahr, A., 2011. Skin penetration and deposition of carboxyfluorescein and temoporfin from different lipid vesicular systems: in vitro study with finite and infinite dosage application. *Int. J. Pharm.* 408(1–2), 223–234.

Chen, H., Zhu, H., Zheng, J., Mou, D., Wan, J., Zhang, J., et al., 2009. Iontophoresis-driven penetration of nanovesicles through microneedle-induced skin microchannels for enhancing transdermal delivery of insulin. *J. Control Release.* 139(1), 63–72.

Chen, J., Jiang, Q.D., Chai, Y.P., Zhang, H., Peng, P., Yang, X.X., 2016. *Natural Terpenes as Penetration Enhancers for Transdermal Drug Delivery.* Vol. 21, Molecules. MDPI AG.

Chourasia, M.K., Kang, L., Chan, S.Y., 2011. Nanosized ethosomes bearing ketoprofen for improved transdermal delivery. *Results Pharma. Sci.* 1(1), 60–67.

Cornwell, P.A., Barry, B.W., 1994 Apr 1. Sesquiterpene Components of Volatile Oils as Skin Penetration Enhancers for the Hydrophilic Permeant 5-Fluorouracil. *J. Pharm. Pharmacol.* 46(4), 261–269.

Cornwell, P.A., Barry, B.W., Stoddart, C.P., Bouwstra, J.A., 1994. Wide-angle X-ray diffraction of human stratum corneum: effects of hydration and terpene enhancer treatment. *J. Pharm. Pharmacol.* 46(12), 938–950.

Cornwell, P.A., Barry, B.W., Bouwstra, J.A., Gooris, G.S., 1996 Jan 15. Modes of action of terpene penetration enhancers in human skin; differential scanning calorimetry, small-angle X-ray diffraction and enhancer uptake studies. *Int. J. Pharm.* 127(1), 9–26.

Cui, Y., Li, L., Zhang, L., Li, J., Gu, J., Gong, H., et al., 2011 Sep. Enhancement and mechanism of transdermal absorption of terpene-induced propranolol hydrochloride. *Arch. Pharm. Res.* 34(9), 1477–1485.

Date, A.A., Srivastava, D., Nagarsenker, M.S., Mulherkar, R., Panicker, L., Aswal, V., et al., 2011 Oct 25. Lecithin-based novel cationic nanocarriers (LeciPlex) I: fabrication, characterization and evaluation. *Nanomedicine* 6(8), 1309–1325.

Dong, P., Teutloff, C., Lademann, J., Patzelt, A., Schäfer-Korting, M., Meinke, M.C., 2020 Jun 1. Solvent effects on skin penetration and spatial distribution of the hydrophilic nitroxide spin probe PCA investigated by EPR. *Cell Biochem. Biophys.* 78(2), 127–137.

Dragicevic, N., Maibach, H.I., 2016. *Percutaneous Penetration Enhancers – Chemical Methods in Penetration Enhancement: Nanocarriers.* Percutaneous Penetration Enhancers – Chemical Methods in Penetration Enhancement: Nanocarriers.

Dragicevic, N., Verma, D.D., Fahr, A., 2016. Invasomes: Vesicles for Enhanced Skin Delivery of Drugs. In: *Percutaneous Penetration Enhancers Chemical Methods in Penetration Enhancement,* Nanocarriers: Springer Berlin Heidelberg, pp. 77–92.

Dragicevic-Curic, N., Fahr, A., 2012. Liposomes in topical photodynamic therapy. *Expert Opin. Drug Deliv.* 9, 1015–1032.

Dragicevic-Curic, N., Scheglmann, D., Albrecht, V., Fahr, A.. 2008 Temoporfin-loaded invasomes: development, characterization and in vitro skin penetration studies. *J. Control Release,* 127(1), 59–69.

Dragicevic-Curic, N., Gräfe, S., Albrecht, V., Fahr, A., 2008. Topical application of temoporfin-loaded invasomes for photodynamic therapy of subcutaneously implanted tumours in mice: a pilot study. *J. Photochem. Photobiol. B Biol.* 91(1), 41–50.

Dragicevic-Curic, N., Scheglmann, D., Albrecht, V., Fahr, A., 2009. Development of different temoporfin-loaded invasomes-novel nanocarriers of temoporfin: characterization, stability and in vitro skin penetration studies. *Colloids Surf. B Biointerfaces.* 70(2), 198–206.

Dragicevic-Curic, N., Scheglmann, D., Albrecht, V., Fahr, A., 2009. Development of liposomes containing ethanol for skin delivery of temoporfin: characterization and in vitro penetration studies. *Colloids Surf. B Biointerfaces.* 74(1), 114–122.

Dragicevic-Curic, N., Gräfe, S., Gitter, B., Fahr, A., 2010. Efficacy of temoporfin-loaded invasomes in the photodynamic therapy in human epidermoid and colorectal tumour cell lines. *J. Photochem. Photobiol. B Biol.* 101(3), 238–250.

Dragicevic-Curic, N., Gräfe, S., Gitter, B., Fahr, A., Winter, S., Fahr, A., et al., 2010. Development of liposomes containing ethanol for skin delivery of temoporfin: characterization and in vitro penetration studies. *Colloids Surf. B Biointerfaces.* 384(1–2), 100–108.

Dragicevic-Curic, N., Friedrich, M., Petersen, S., Scheglmann, D., Douroumis, D., Plass, W., et al., 2011 Jun 30. Assessment of fluidity of different invasomes by electron spin resonance and differential scanning calorimetry. *Int. J. Pharm.* 412(1–2), 85–94.

Duangjit, S., Nimcharoenwan, T., Chomya, N., Locharoenrat, N., Ngawhirunpat, T., 2016. Design and development of optimal invasomes for transdermal drug delivery using computer program. *Asian J. Pharm. Sci.* 11(1), 52–53.

Dubey, V., Mishra, D., Dutta, T., Nahar, M., Saraf, D.K., Jain, N.K., 2007 Nov 6. Dermal and transdermal delivery of an anti-psoriatic agent via ethanolic liposomes. *J. Control Release.* 123(2), 148–154.

Dul, M., Stefanidou, M., Porta, P., Serve, J., O'Mahony, C., Malissen, B., et al., 2017 Nov 10. Hydrodynamic gene delivery in human skin using a hollow microneedle device. *J. Control Release.* 265, 120–131.

Dwivedi, M., Sharma, V., Pathak, K., 2017 Feb 1. Pilosebaceous targeting by isotretenoin-loaded invasomal gel for the treatment of eosinophilic pustular folliculitis: optimization, efficacy and cellular analysis. *Drug Dev. Ind. Pharm.* 43(2), 293–304.

El Maghraby, G.M., Williams, A.C., 2009. Vesicular systems for delivering conventional small organic molecules and larger macromolecules to and through human skin. *Expert Opin. Drug Deliv.* 6, 149–163.

El Maghraby, G.M.M., Williams, A.C., Barry, B.W., 1999 Oct. Skin delivery of oestradiol from deformable and traditiona liposomes: mechanistic studies. *J. Pharm. Pharmacol.* 51(10), 1123–1134.

El Maghraby, G.M.M., Williams, A.C., Barry, B.W., 2001 Oct. Skin hydration and possible shunt route penetration in controlled estradiol delivery from ultradeformable and standard liposomes. *J. Pharm. Pharmacol.* 53(10), 1311–1322.

El-Kattan, A.F., Asbill, C.S., Michniak, B.B., 2000. The effect of terpene enhancer lipophilicity on the percutaneous permeation of hydrocortisone formulated in HPMC gel systems. *Int. J. Pharm.* 198(2), 179–189.

El-Kattan, A.F., Asbill, C.S., Kim, N., Michniak, B.B., 2001 Mar 14. The effects of terpene enhancers on the percutaneous permeation of drugs with different lipophilicities. *Int. J. Pharm.* 215(1–2), 229–240.

El-Nabarawi, M.A., Shamma, R.N., Farouk, F., Nasralla, S.M., 2018. Dapsone-loaded invasomes as a potential treatment of acne: preparation, characterization, and in vivo skin deposition assay. *AAPS Pharm. Sci. Tech.* 19(5), 2174–2184.

Elsabahy, M., Foldvari, M., 2013 Dec 31. Needle-free gene delivery through the skin: an overview of recent strategies. *Curr. Pharm. Des.* 19(41), 7301–7315.

Erdal, M.S., Peköz, A.Y., Aksu, B., Araman, A., 2014. Impacts of chemical enhancers on skin permeation and deposition of terbinafine. *Pharm. Dev. Technol.* 19(5), 565–570.

Escobar-Chávez, J.J., Bonilla-Martínez, D., Villegas-González, M.A., Revilla-Vázquez, A.L., 2009 Nov. Electroporation as an efficient physical enhancer for skin drug delivery. *J. Clin. Pharmacol.* 49(11), 1262–1283.

Fang, J.Y., Yu, S.Y., Wu, P.C., Huang, Y Bin, Tsai, Y.H., 2001. In vitro skin permeation of estradiol from various proniosome formulations. *Int. J. Pharm.* 215(1–2), 91–99.

Fluhr, J.W., Berardesca, E., 2000. Effects of Moisturizers and Keratolytic Agents in Psoriasis. In: Loden, M., Maibach, H.I. (eds) *Dry Skin and Moisturizers Chemistry and Function.* Boca Raton, London, New York, pp. 167–172.

Gao, S., Singh, J., 1998. In vitro percutaneous absorption enhancement of a lipophilic drug tamoxifen by terpenes. *J. Control Release.* 51(2–3), 193–199.

Garcia-Manyes, S., Oncins, G., Sanz, F., 2006 Jul 15. Effect of pH and ionic strength on phospholipid nanomechanics and on deposition process onto hydrophilic surfaces measured by AFM. *Electrochim. Acta.* 51(24), 5029–5036.

Garg, B.J., Garg, N.K., Beg, S., Singh, B., Katare, O.P., 2016 Mar 15. Nanosized ethosomes-based hydrogel formulations of methoxsalen for enhanced topical delivery against vitiligo: formulation optimization, in vitro evaluation and preclinical assessment. *J. Drug Target.* 24(3), 233–246.

Ghafourian, T., Zandasrar, P., Hamishekar, H., Nokhodchi, A., 2004. The effect of penetration enhancers on drug delivery through skin: a QSAR study. *J. Control Release.* 99(1), 113–125.

Goates, C.Y., Knutson, K., 1994. Enhanced permeation of polar compounds through human epidermis. I. Permeability and membrane structural changes in the presence of short chain alcohols. *BBA – Biomembr.* 1195(1), 169–179.

Godin, B., Touitou, E., 2003. Ethosomes: new prospects in transdermal delivery. *Crit. Rev. Ther. Drug Carrier Syst.* 20,63–102.

Gomaa, Y.A., El-Khordagui, L.K., Garland, M.J., Donnelly, R.F., McInnes, F., Meidan, V.M., 2012. Effect of microneedle treatment on the skin permeation of a nanoencapsulated dye. *J. Pharm. Pharmacol.* 64(11), 1592–1602.

Haag, S.F., Fleige, E., Chen, M., Fahr, A., Teutloff, C., Bittl, R., et al., 2011. Skin penetration enhancement of core-multishell nanotransporters and invasomes measured by electron paramagnetic resonance spectroscopy. *Int. J. Pharm.* 416(1), 223–228.

Hao, Y., Li, W., Zhou, X.L., Yang, F., Qian, Z.Y., 2017. Microneedles-based transdermal drug delivery systems: a review. *J. Biomed. Nanotechnol.* 13, 1581–1597.

Hatta, I., Nakazawa, H., Obata, Y., Ohta, N., Inoue, K., Yagi, N., 2010. Novel method to observe subtle structural modulation of stratum corneum on applying chemical agents. *Chem. Phys. Lipids.* 163(4–5), 381–389.

Heard, C.M., Kung, D., Thomas, C.P., 2006. Skin penetration enhancement of mefenamic acid by ethanol and 1,8-cineole can be explained by the "pull" effect. *Int. J. Pharm.* 321(1–2), 167–170.

Hofland, H.E.J., van der Geest, R., Bodde, H.E., Junginger, H.E., Bouwstra, J.A., 1994. Estradiol permeation from nonionic surfactant vesicles through human stratum corneum in vitro. *Pharm. Res. Off. J. Am. Assoc. Pharm. Sci.* 11(5), 659–664.

Honeywell-Nguyen, P.L., Frederik, P.M., Bomans, P.H.H., Junginger, H.E., Bouwstra, J.A., 2002. Transdermal delivery of pergolide from surfactant-based elastic and rigid vesicles: characterization and in vitro transport studies. *Pharm. Res.* 19(7), 991–997.

Hoppel, M., Baurecht, D., Holper, E., Mahrhauser, D., Valenta, C., 2014 Sep 10. Validation of the combined ATR-FTIR/tape stripping technique for monitoring the distribution of surfactants in the stratum corneum. *Int. J. Pharm.* 472(1–2), 88–93.

Hori, M., Satoh, S., Maibach, H.I., Guy, R.H., 1991. Enhancement of propranolol hydrochloride and diazepam skin absorption in vitro: effect of enhancer lipophilicity. *J. Pharm. Sci.* 80(1), 32–35.

Jaimes-Lizcano, Y.A., Lawson, L.B., Papadopoulos, K.D., 2011. Oil-frozen W1/O/W2 double emulsions for dermal biomacromolecular delivery containing ethanol as chemical penetration enhancer. *J. Pharm. Sci.* 100(4), 1398–1406.

Jain, A.K., Thomas, N.S., Panchagnula, R., 2002 Feb 19. Transdermal drug delivery of imipramine hydrochloride. I. Effect of terpenes. *J. Control Release.* 79(1–3), 93–101.

Jamaledin, R., Di Natale, C., Onesto, V., Taraghdari, Z.B., Zare, E.N., Makvandi, P., et al., 2020 Feb 17. Progress in microneedle-mediated protein delivery. *J. Clin. Med.* 9(2), 542.

Joo, H.H., Kim, J.C., Lee, H.Y., 2008. In vitro permeation study of hinokitiol: effects of vehicles and enhancers. *Drug Deliv.* 15(1), 19–22.

Kadir, R.O.N., Stempler, D.O.V., 1987. Alkanoic acid solutions: a "push-pull" mechanism. 76(10), 1–6.

Kalpana, B., Lakshmi, P.K., 2013. Transdermal permeation enhancement of Tolterodine Tartrate through invasomes and iontophoresis. *Der. Pharm. Lett.* 5(6), 119–126.

Kaltschmidt, B.P., Ennen, I., Greiner, J.F.W., Dietsch, R., Patel, A., Kaltschmidt, B., et al., 2020 May 1. Preparation of terpenoid-invasomes with selective activity against S. aureus and characterization by cryo transmission electron microscopy. *Biomedicines* 8(5), 105.

Kamran, M., Ahad, A., Aqil, M., Imam, S.S., Sultana, Y., Ali, A., 2016. Design, formulation and optimization of novel soft nano-carriers for transdermal olmesartan medoxomil delivery: in vitro characterization and in vivo pharmacokinetic assessment. *Int. J. Pharm.* 505(1–2), 147–158.

Kearney, M.C., Caffarel-Salvador, E., Fallows, S.J., McCarthy, H.O., Donnelly, R.F., 2016 Jun 1. Microneedle-mediated delivery of donepezil: potential for improved treatment options in Alzheimer's disease. *Eur. J. Pharm. Biopharm.* 103, 43–50.

Kelbauskas, L., 2003. *Untersuchungen zur Struktur-Eigenschafts-Beziehung selbstassoziierender Photosensibilisatoren mittels zeitaufgelöster Spektroskopie.* Friedrich-Schiller Univ Jena, Jena, PhD Thesis.

Khan, M.A., Pandit, J., Sultana, Y., Sultana, S., Ali, A., Aqil, M., et al., 2015 Aug 18. Novel carbopol-based transfersomal gel of 5-fluorouracil for skin cancer treatment: *in vitro* characterization and *in vivo* study. *Drug Deliv.* 22(6), 795–802.

Kirjavainen, M., Urtti, A., Valjakka-Koskela, R., Kiesvaara, J., Mönkkönen, J., 1999 Mar 1. Liposome-skin interactions and their effects on the skin permeation of drugs. *Eur. J. Pharm. Sci.* 7(4), 279–286.

Kirjavainen, M., Urtti, A., Jääskeläinen, I., Marjukka Suhonen, T., Paronen, P., Valjakka-Koskela, R., et al., 1996 Dec 13. Interaction of liposomes with human skin in vitro – The influence of lipid composition and structure. *Biochim. Biophys. Acta – Lipids Lipid Metab.* 1304(3), 179–189.

Kirjavainen, M., Mönkkönen, J., Saukkosaari, M., Valjakka-Koskela, R., Kiesvaara, J., Urtti, A., 1999 Mar 29. Phospholipids affect stratum corneum lipid bilayer fluidity and drug partitioning into the bilayers. *J. Control Release.* 58(2), 207–214.

Korting, H.C., Schäfer-Korting, M., 2010. *Carriers in the topical treatment of skin disease.* Vol. 197, Handbook of Experimental Pharmacology. Handb Exp Pharmacol. pp. 435–468.

Krishnaiah,, Y.S., Bhaskar,, P., Satyanarayana,, V., 2004. Penetration-enhancing effect of ethanol-water solvent system and ethanolic solution of carvone on transdermal permeability of nimodipine from HPMC gel across rat abdominal skin. *Pharm. Dev. Technol.* 9(1), 63–74.

Krishnaiah, Y.S.R., Satyanarayana, V., Bhaskar, P., 2003. Enhanced percutaneous permeability of nicardipine hydrochloride by carvone across the rat abdominal skin. *Drug Dev. Ind. Pharm.* 29(2), 191–202.

Krishnaiah, Y.S.R., Al-Saidan, S.M., Chandrasekhar, D.V., Rama, B., 2006. Effect of nerodilol and carvone on in vitro permeation of nicorandil across rat epidermal membrane. *Drug Dev. Ind. Pharm.* 32(4), 423–435.

Kübler, A.C., Haase, T., Staff, C., Kahle, B., Rheinwald, M., Mühling, J., 1999. Photodynamic therapy of primary nonmelanomatous skin tumours of the head and neck. *Lasers Surg. Med.* 25(1), 60–68.

Kunta, J.R., Goskonda, V.R., Brotherton, H.O., Khan, M.A., Reddy, I.K., 1997. Effect of menthol and related terpenes on the percutaneous absorption of propranolol across excised hairless mouse skin. *J. Pharm. Sci.* 86(12), 1369–1373.

Kurihara-Bergstrom, T., Knutson, K., DeNoble, L.J., Goates, C.Y., 1990. Percutaneous absorption enhancement of an ionic molecule by ethanol–water systems in human skin. *Pharm. Res. Off. J. Am. Assoc. Pharm. Sci.* 7(7), 762–766.

Lakshmi, P., Lakshmi, P.K., Mounica, V., Manoj, K.Y., Prasanthi, D., 2014 Jun 21. Preparation and evaluation of curcumin invasomes. *Int. J. Drug Deliv.* 6(2), 113–120.

Lan, Y., Li, H., Chen, Y yan, Zhang, Y wen, Liu, N., Zhang, Q., et al., 2014. Essential oil from Zanthoxylum bungeanum Maxim and its main components used as transdermal penetration enhancers: a comparative study. *J. Zhejiang Univ. Sci. B.* 15(11), 940–952.

Lan, Y., Wang, J., Li, H., Zhang, Y., Chen, Y., Zhao, B., et al., 2016 May 18. Effect of menthone and related compounds on skin permeation of drugs with different lipophilicity and molecular organization of stratum corneum lipids. *Pharm. Dev. Technol.* 21(4), 389–398.

Lee, S.E., Seo, J., Lee, S.H., 2017. The mechanism of sonophoresis and the penetration pathways. In: *Percutaneous Penetration Enhancers Physical Methods in Penetration Enhancement*. Springer Berlin Heidelberg. p. 15–30.

Levison, K.K., Takayama, K., Isowa, K., Okabe, K., Nagai, T., 1994. Formulation optimization of indomethacin gels containing a combination of three kinds of cyclic monoterpenes as percutaneous penetration enhancers. *J. Pharm. Sci.* 83(9), 1367–1372.

Liu, H., Li, S., Wang, Y., Yao, H., Zhang, Y., 2006 Mar 27. Effect of vehicles and enhancers on the topical delivery of cyclosporin A. *Int. J. Pharm.* 311(1–2), 182–186.

Loan Honeywell-Nguyen, P., De Graaff, A.M., Wouter Groenink, H.W., Bouwstra, J.A., 2002 Nov 14. The in vivo and in vitro interactions of elastic and rigid vesicles with human skin. *Biochim. Biophys. Acta - Gen. Subj.* 1573(2), 130–140.

Makino, K., Yamada, T., Kimura, M., Oka, T., Ohshima, H., Kondo, T., 1991. Temperature- and ionic strength-induced conformational changes in the lipid head group region of liposomes as suggested by zeta potential data. *Biophys. Chem.* 41(2), 175–183.

McAlister, E., Garland, M.J., Singh, T.R.R., Donnelly, R.F., 2017. Microporation using microneedle arrays. In: *Percutaneous Penetration Enhancers Physical Methods in Penetration Enhancement*. Springer Berlin Heidelberg, pp. 273–303.

Megrab, N.A., Williams, A.C., Barry, B.W., 1995. Oestradiol permeation across human skin, silastic and snake skin membranes: the effects of ethanol/water co-solvent systems. *Int. J. Pharm.* 116(1), 101–112.

Mitragotri, S., 2017. Sonophoresis: Ultrasound-mediated transdermal drug delivery. In: *Percutaneous Penetration Enhancers Physical Methods in Penetration Enhancement*. Springer Berlin Heidelberg. p. 3–14.

Moghimi, H.R., Williams, A.C., Barry, B.W., 1997 Jan 1. A lamellar matrix model for stratum corneum intercellular lipids. V. Effects of terpene penetration enhancers on the structure and thermal behaviour of the matrix. *Int. J. Pharm.* 146(1), 41–54.

Monti, D., Saettone, M.F., Giannaccini, B., Galli-Angeli, D., 1995 Jan 1. Enhancement of transdermal penetration of dapiprazole through hairless mouse skin. *J. Control Release.* 33(1), 71–77.

Monti, D., Chetoni, P., Burgalassi, S., Najarro, M., Saettone, M.F., Boldrini, E., 2002. Effect of different terpene-containing essential oils on permeation of estradiol through hairless mouse skin. *Int. J. Pharm.* 237(1–2), 209–214.

Morimoto, Y., Wada, Y., Seki, T., Sugibayashi, K., 2002. In vitro skin permeation of morphine hydrochloride during the finite application of penetration-enhancing system containing water, ethanol and l-menthol. *Biol. Pharm. Bull.* 25(1), 134–136.

Morimoto, Y., Hayashi, T., Kawabata, S., Seki, T., Sugibayashi, K., 2000 Oct 1. Effect of l-menthol-ethanol-water system on the systemic absorption of Flurbiprofen after repeated topical applications in rabbits. *Biol. Pharm. Bull.* 23(10), 1254–1257.

Mura, S., Manconi, M., Sinico, C., Valenti, D., Fadda, A.M., 2009. Penetration enhancer-containing vesicles (PEVs) as carriers for cutaneous delivery of minoxidil. *Int. J. Pharm.* 380(1–2), 72–79.

Mutalik, S., Parekh, H.S., Davies, N.M., Udupa, N., 2009 Feb. A combined approach of chemical enhancers and sonophoresis for the transdermal delivery of tizanidine hydrochloride. *Drug Deliv.* 16(2), 82–91.

Narishetty, S.T.K., Panchagnula, R., 2004. Transdermal delivery of zidovudine: effect of terpenes and their mechanism of action. *J. Control Release.* 95(3), 367–379.

Narishetty, S.T.K., Panchagnula, R., 2005. Effect of L-menthol and 1,8-cineole on phase behavior and molecular organization of SC lipids and skin permeation of zidovudine. *J. Control Release.* 102(1), 59–70.

Ntimenou, V., Fahr, A., Antimisiaris, S.G., 2012. Elastic vesicles for transdermal drug delivery of hydrophilic drugs: a comparison of important physicochemical characteristics of different vesicle types. *J. Biomed. Nanotechnol.* 8(4), 613–623.

Nokhodchi,, A., Sharabiani,, K., Rashidi,, M.R., Ghafourian,, T., 2007. The effect of terpene concentrations on the skin penetration of diclofenac sodium. *Int. J. Pharm.* 335(1–2), 97–105.

Obata, Y., Takayama, K., Machida, Y., Nagai, T., 1991 Dec 1. Combined effect of cyclic monoterpenes and ethanol on percutaneous absorption of diclofenac sodium. *Drug Des. Discov.* 8(2), 137–144.

Obata, Y., Utsumi, S., Watanabe, H., Suda, M., Tokudome, Y., Otsuka, M., et al., 2010. Infrared spectroscopic study of lipid interaction in stratum corneum treated with transdermal absorption enhancers. *Int. J. Pharm.* 389(1–2), 18–23.

Ogiso, T., Iwaki, M., Paku, T., 1995. Effect of various enhancers on transdermal penetration of indomethacin and urea, and relationship between penetration parameters and enhancement factors. *J. Pharm. Sci.* 84(4), 482–488.

Okabe, H., Takayama, K., Ogura, A., Nagai, T., 1989 Jun 1. Effects of limonene and related compounds on the percutaneous absorption of indomethacin. *Drug Des. Deliv.* 4(4), 313–321.

Okabe, H., Obata, Y., Takayama, K., Nagai, T., 1990 Sep 1. Percutaneous absorption enhancing effect and skin irritation of monocyclic monoterpenes. *Drug Des. Deliv.* 6(3), 229–238.

Ota, Y., Hamada, A., Saito, H., Nakano, M., 2003. Evaluation of Percutaneous Absorption of Midazolam by Terpenes. *Drug Metab. Pharmacokinet.* 18(4), 261–266.

Parikh, D.K., Ghosh, T.K., 2005. Feasibility of transdermal delivery of fluoxetine. *AAPS Pharm. Sci. Tech.* 6(2), 144–149.

Park, J.H., Choi, S.O., Seo, S., Choy, Y Bin, Prausnitz, M.R., 2010 Oct 1. A microneedle roller for transdermal drug delivery. *Eur. J. Pharm. Biopharm.* 76(2), 282–289.

Pershing, L.K., Lambert, L.D., Knutson, K., 1990. Mechanism of ethanol-enhanced estradiol permeation across human skin in vivo. *Pharm. Res. Off. J. Am. Assoc. Pharm. Sci.* 7, 170–175.

Prasanthi, D., K. Lakshmi, P. Iontophoretic,, 2013 Feb 1. Transdermal delivery of finasteride in vesicular invasomal carriers. *Pharm. Nanotechnol.* 1(2), 136–150.

Puglia, C., Bonina, F., Trapani, G., Franco, M., Ricci, M., 2001 Oct 9. Evaluation of in vitro percutaneous absorption of lorazepam and clonazepam from hydroalcoholic gel formulations. *Int. J. Pharm.* 228(1–2), 79–87.

Puri, A., Nguyen, H.X., Banga, A.K., 2016 Oct 1. Microneedle-mediated intradermal delivery of epigallocatechin-3-gallate. *Int. J. Cosmet. Sci.* 38(5), 512–523.

Qadri, G.R., Ahad, A., Aqil, M., Imam, S.S., Ali, A., 2017 Jan 2. Invasomes of isradipine for enhanced transdermal delivery against hypertension: formulation, characterization, and in vivo pharmacodynamic study. *Artif. Cells Nanomed. Biotechnol.* 45(1), 139–145.

Rastogi, R., Anand, S., Koul, V., 2010 Nov. Electroporation of polymeric nanoparticles: an alternative technique for transdermal delivery of insulin. *Drug Dev. Ind. Pharm.* 36(11), 1303–1311.

Rhee, Y.S., Choi, J.G., Park, E.S., Chi, S.C., 2001 Oct 9. Transdermal delivery of ketoprofen using microemulsions. *Int. J. Pharm.* 228(1–2), 161–170.

Rhodes, L.E., 2000. Essential fatty acids. In: Loden, M., Maibach, H.I. *Dry Skin and Moisturizers Chemistry and Function.* Boca Raton, London, New York. pp. 311–325.

Ripolin, A., Quinn, J., Larrañeta, E., Vicente-Perez, E.M., Barry, J., Donnelly, R.F., 2017 Apr 15. Successful application of large microneedle patches by human volunteers. *Int. J. Pharm.* 521(1–2), 92–101.

Rizwan, M., Aqil, M., Ahad, A., Sultana, Y., Ali, M.M., 2008. Transdermal delivery of valsartan: I. Effect of various terpenes. *Drug Dev. Ind. Pharm.* 34(6), 618–626.

Ronnander, J.P., Simon, L., Koch, A., 2019 Nov 1. Transdermal delivery of sumatriptan succinate using iontophoresis and dissolving microneedles. *J. Pharm. Sci.* 108(11), 3649–3656.

Sabri, A.H., Ogilvie, J., Abdulhamid, K., Shpadaruk, V., McKenna, J., Segal, J., et al., 2019. Expanding the applications of microneedles in dermatology. *Eur. J. Pharm. Biopharm.* 140, 121–140.

Sabri, A.H., Kim, Y., Marlow, M., Scurr, D.J., Segal, J., Banga, A.K., et al., 2020. Intradermal and transdermal drug delivery using microneedles – fabrication, performance evaluation and application to lymphatic delivery. *Advanced Drug Delivery Reviews.* Elsevier B.V.

Saffari, M., Shirazi, H., Moghimi, H.R., 2016. *Terpene-loaded Liposomes and Isopropyl Myristate as Chemical Permeation Enhancers Toward Liposomal Gene Delivery in Lung Cancer cells; A Comparative Study.* Vol. 15, Shaheed Beheshti University of Medical Sciences and Health Services Iranian Journal of Pharmaceutical Research.

Sala, M., Diab, R., Elaissari, A., Fessi, H., 2018. Lipid nanocarriers as skin drug delivery systems: properties, mechanisms of skin interactions and medical applications. *Int. J. Pharm.* 535(1–2), 1–17.

Sammeta, S.M., Repka, M.A., Murthy, S.N., 2011 Sep. Magnetophoresis in combination with chemical enhancers for transdermal drug delivery. *Drug Dev. Ind. Pharm.* 37(9), 1076–1082.

Sapra, B., Jain, S., Tiwary, A.K., 2008. Percutaneous permeation enhancement by terpenes: mechanistic view. *AAPS J.*10, 120–132.

Shah, D.K., Khandavilli, S., Panchagnula, R., 2008 Sep. Alteration of skin hydration and its barrier function by vehicle and permeation enhancers: a study using TGA, FTIR, TEWL and drug permeation as markers. *Methods Find Exp. Clin. Pharmacol.* 30(7), 499–512.

Shah, S.M., Ashtikar, M., Jain, A.S., Makhija, D.T., Nikam, Y., Gude, R.P., et al., 2015. LeciPlex, invasomes, and liposomes: a skin penetration study. *Int. J. Pharm.* 490(1–2), 391–403.

Shamma, R.N., Sayed, S., Sabry, N.A., El-Samanoudy, S.I., 2019 Jul 3. Enhanced skin targeting of retinoic acid spanlastics: in vitro characterization and clinical evaluation in acne patients. *J. Liposome Res.* 29(3), 283–290.

Sharma, V., Yusuf, M., Pathak, K., 2014. Nanovesicles for transdermal delivery of felodipine: development, characterization, and pharmacokinetics. *Int. J. Pharm. Investig.* 4(3), 119.

Sharma, G., Goyal, H., Thakur, K., Raza, K., Katare, O.P., 2016 Oct 12. Novel elastic membrane vesicles (EMVs) and ethosomes-mediated effective topical delivery of aceclofenac: a new therapeutic approach for pain and inflammation. *Drug Deliv.* 23(8), 3135–3145.

Sieber, M.A., Hegel, J.K.E., 2013 Nov. Azelaic acid: properties and mode of action. *Skin Pharmacol. Physiol.* 27(SUPPL.1), 9–17.

Singh, P., Carrier, A., Chen, Y., Lin, S., Wang, J., Cui, S., et al., 2019. Polymeric microneedles for controlled transdermal drug delivery. *J. Controlled Release* 315, 97–113.

Song, Y.K., Kim, C.K., 2006. Topical delivery of low-molecular-weight heparin with surface-charged flexible liposomes. *Biomaterials* 27(2), 271–280.

Songkro,, S., Rades,, T., Becket,, G., 2009. Effects of some terpenes on the in vitro permeation of LHRH through newborn pig skin. *Pharmazie.* 64(2), 110–115.

Tas, C., Ozkan, Y., Okyar, A., Savaser, A., 2007. In vitro and ex vivo permeation studies of etodolac from hydrophilic gels and effect of terpenes as enhancers. *Drug Deliv.* 14(7), 453–459.

Tawfik, M.A., Ibrahim, M., Magdy, T., Mohamed, I., Nageeb El-Helaly, S., 2020. Low-frequency versus high-frequency ultrasound-mediated transdermal delivery of agomelatine-loaded invasomes: development, optimization and in-vivo pharmacokinetic assessment. *Int. J. Nanomedicine.* 15, 8893–8910. doi: 10.2147/IJN.S283911.

Thoma, K., Jocham, U.E., 1992. Liposome Dermatics: Assessment of Long-Term Stability. In: *Liposome Dermatics.* Springer Berlin Heidelberg. pp. 150–166.

Thomas, N.S., Panchagnula, R., 2003. Transdermal delivery of zidovudine: effect of vehicles on permeation across rat skin and their mechanism of action. *Eur. J. Pharm. Sci.* 18(1), 71–79.

Touitou, E., Dayan, N., Bergelson, L., Godin, B., Eliaz, M., 2000 Apr 3. Ethosomes - Novel vesicular carriers for enhanced delivery: characterization and skin penetration properties. *J. Control Release.* 65(3), 403–418.

Trauer, S., Richter, H., Kuntsche, J., Büttemeyer, R., Liebsch, M., Linscheid, M., et al., 2014. Influence of massage and occlusion on the ex vivo skin penetration of rigid liposomes and invasomes. *Eur. J. Pharm. Biopharm.* 86(2), 301–306.

Vaddi, H.K., Ho, P.C., Chan, S.Y., 2002. Terpenes in propylene glycol as skin-penetration enhancers: permeation and partition of haloperidol, fourier transform infrared spectroscopy, and differential scanning calorimetry. *J. Pharm. Sci.* 91(7), 1639–1651.

Vaddi, H.K., Ho, P.C., Chan, Y.W., Chan, S.Y., 2002. Terpenes in ethanol: haloperidol permeation and partition through human skin and stratum corneum changes. *J. Control Release.* 81(1–2), 121–133.

Van Den Bergh, B.A.I., Vroom, J., Gerritsen, H., Junginger, H.E., Bouwstra, J.A., 1999. Interactions of elastic and rigid vesicles with human skin in vitro: electron microscopy and two-photon excitation microscopy. *Biochim. Biophys. Acta – Biomembr.* 1461(1), 155–173.

Van Kuijk-Meuwissen, M.E.M.J., Junginger, H.E., Bouwstra, J.A., 1998. Interactions between liposomes and human skin in vitro, a confocal laser scanning microscopy study. *Biochim. Biophys. Acta – Biomembr.* 1371(1), 31–39.

Van Kuijk-Meuwissen, M.E.M.J., Mougin, L., Junginger, H.E., Bouwstra, J.A., 1998. Application of vesicles to rat skin in vivo: a confocal laser scanning microscopy study. *J. Control Release.* 56(1–3), 189–196.

Verma, D.D., 2002. *Invasomes-Novel Topical Carriers for Enhanced Topical Delivery: Characterization and Skin Penetration Properties.* Philipps-University Marburg, Germany

Verma, D.D., Fahr, A., 2004. Synergistic penetration enhancement effect of ethanol and phospholipids on the topical delivery of cyclosporin a. *J. Control Release.* 97(1), 55–66.

Verma, D.D., Verma, S., Blume, G., Fahr, A., 2003. Liposomes increase skin penetration of entrapped and non-entrapped hydrophilic substances into human skin: a skin penetration and confocal laser scanning microscopy study. *Eur. J. Pharm. Biopharm.* 55(3), 271–277.

Verma, D.D., Verma, S., Blume, G., Fahr, A., 2003. Particle size of liposomes influences dermal delivery of substances into skin. *Int. J. Pharm.* 258(1–2), 141–151.

Verma, D.D., Verma, S., McElwee, K.J., Freyschmidt-Paul, P., Hoffman, R., Fahr, A., 2004. Treatment of alopecia areata in the DEBR model using Cyclosporin A lipid vesicles. *Eur. J. Dermatol.* 14(5), 332–338.

Vicente-Perez, E.M., Larrañeta, E., McCrudden, M.T.C., Kissenpfennig, A., Hegarty, S., McCarthy, H.O., et al., 2017 Aug 1. Repeat application of microneedles does not alter skin appearance or barrier function and causes no measurable disturbance of serum biomarkers of infection, inflammation or immunity in mice in vivo. *Eur. J. Pharm. Biopharm.* 117, 400–407.

Vidya, K., Lakshmi, P.K., 2019. Cytotoxic effect of transdermal invasomal anastrozole gel on MCF-7 breast cancer cell line. *J. Appl. Pharm. Sci.* 9(03), 50–058.

Waller, J.M., Dreher, F., Behnam, S., Ford, C., Lee, C., Tiet, T., et al., 2006 Aug. 'Keratolytic' properties of benzoyl peroxide and retinoic acid resemble salicylic acid in man. *Skin Pharmacol. Physiol.* 19(5), 283–289.

Wang, J., Dong, C., Song, Z., Zhang, W., He, X., Zhang, R., et al., 2017 May 19. Monocyclic monoterpenes as penetration enhancers of ligustrazine hydrochloride for dermal delivery. *Pharm. Dev. Technol.* 22(4), 571–577.

Watanabe, H., Obata, Y., Ishida, K., Takayama, K., 2009. Effect of l-menthol on the thermotropic behavior of ceramide 2/cholesterol mixtures as a model for the intercellular lipids in stratum corneum. *Colloids Surf. B Biointerfaces.* 73(1), 116–121.

Wempe, M.F., Lightner, J.W., Zoeller, E.L., Rice, P.J., 2009 Mar 1. Investigating idebenone and idebenone linoleate metabolism: *in vitro* pig ear and mouse melanocyte studies. *J. Cosmet Dermatol.* 8(1), 63–73.

Williams, A.C., Barry, B.W., 1989. Permeation, FTIR and DSC investigations of terpene penetration enhancers in human skin. *J. Pharm. Pharmacol.* 41(Suppl), 12P.

Williams, A.C., Barry, B.W., 1991a. Terpenes and the lipid–protein–partitioning theory of skin penetration enhancement. *Pharm. Res. Off. J. Am Assoc. Pharm. Sci.* 8(1), 17–24.

Williams, A.C., Barry, B.W., 1991b. The enhancement index concept applied to terpene penetration enhancers for human skin and model lipophilic (oestradiol) and hydrophilic (5-fluorouracil) drugs. *Int. J. Pharm.* 74(2–3), 157–168.

Williams, A.C., Barry, B.W., 2004. Penetration enhancers. *Adv. Drug Deliv. Rev.* 56(5), 603–618.

Xie, F., Chai, J.K., Hu, Q., Yu, Y.H., Ma, L., Liu, L.Y., et al., 2016 Jun 30. Transdermal permeation of drugs with differing lipophilicity: effect of penetration enhancer camphor. *Int. J. Pharm.* 507(1–2), 90–101.

Yamane, M.A., Williams, A.C., Barry, B.W., 1995. Terpene penetration enhancers in propylene glycol/water co-solvent systems: effectiveness and mechanism of action. *J. Pharm. Pharmacol.* 47(12 A), 978–989.

Yamato, K., Takahashi, Y., Akiyama, H., Tsuji, K., Onishi, H., Machida, Y., 2009. Effect of penetration enhancers on transdermal delivery of propofol. *Biol. Pharm. Bull.* 32(4), 677–683.

Yang, Z., Teng, Y., Wang, H., Hou, H., 2013 Apr 15. Enhancement of skin permeation of bufalin by limonene via reservoir type transdermal patch: formulation design and biopharmaceutical evaluation. *Int. J. Pharm.* 447(1–2), 231–240.

Ye, Y., Yu, J., Wen, D., Kahkoska, A.R., Gu, Z., 2018. Polymeric microneedles for transdermal protein delivery. *Adv. Drug Deliv. Rev.* 127, 106–118.

Yi, Q.F., Yan, J., Tang, S.Y., Huang, H., Kang, L.Y., 2016 Jul 2. Effect of borneol on the transdermal permeation of drugs with differing lipophilicity and molecular organization of stratum corneum lipids. *Drug Dev. Ind. Pharm.* 42(7), 1086–1093.

Yokomizo, Y., Sagitani, H., 1996a. Effects of phospholipids on the in vitro percutaneous penetration of prednisolone and analysis of mechanism by using attenuated total reflectance- Fourier transform infrared spectroscopy. *J. Pharm. Sci.* 85(11), 1220–1226.

Yokomizo, Y., Sagitani, H., 1996b Feb 1. Effects of phospholipids on the percutaneous penetration of indomethacin through the dorsal skin of guinea pigs in vitro. *J. Control Release.* 38(2–3), 267–274.

Zellmer, S., Pfeil, W., Lasch, J., 1995 Jul 26. Interaction of phosphatidylcholine liposomes with the human stratum corneum. *BBA – Biomembr.* 1237(2), 176–182.

Zhai, Y., Xu, R., Wang, Y., Liu, J., Wang, Z., Zhai, G., 2015 Oct 2. Ethosomes for skin delivery of ropivacaine: preparation, characterization and ex vivo penetration properties. *J. Liposome Res.* 25(4), 316–324.

Zhao, K., Singh, J., 1998 Nov 13. Mechanisms of percutaneous absorption of tamoxifen by terpenes: eugenol, D-limonene and menthone. *J. Control Release.* 55(2–3), 253–260.

Zhao, K., Singh, J., 1999 Dec 6. In vitro percutaneous absorption enhancement of propranolol hydrochloride through porcine epidermis by terpenes/ethanol. *J. Control Release.* 62(3), 359–366.

Zhao, K., Singh, S., Singh, J., 2001. Effect of menthone on the in vitro percutaneous absorption of tamoxifen and skin reversibility. *Int. J. Pharm.* 219(1–2), 177–181.

Zhou, W., He, S., Yang, Y., Jian, D., Chen, X., Ding, J., 2015 Jul 1. Formulation, characterization and clinical evaluation of propranolol hydrochloride gel for transdermal treatment of superficial infantile hemangioma. *Drug Dev. Ind. Pharm.* 41(7), 1109–1119.

Index

Note: *Italicized* page numbers refer to figures, **bold** page numbers refer to tables

accelerants, 19–21
acne vulgaris, 44, **49**, 56, 57, 158–159,
    176–178
acyclovir, **75**
acyclovir palmitate, **75**
adapalene, **49**
agomelatine, 124, 125, 128, 129
alcohols, 112, 113, 120, 143
alopecia, **49**, 57, 149, 159–160, 171, *174*
alpha-pinene oxide, 112
amides, 19
5-aminolevulinic acid (5-ALA), **54**, 56
amphotericin B, **55**
anastrozole, 128, 144–145, **173**
anethol, 112, 113
anthralin, **51**
anti-acne drugs, **137**, 158–159, **172**, 177
anti-cancer therapy, 171–176, **172–173**
antigen, **80**
antihypertensive drugs, 152–156
antioxidants, 148
ascorbic acid, **53**
attenuated total reflection-Fourier transform
    infrared spectroscopy (ATR-
    FTIR), 116–118
avanafil, 128, 129, **140**, 160–161, *161*
azelaic acid, 126, **137**, **172**, 176–178, *179*
azithromycin, **46**
Azone, 19, 111, 113, 118

bacitracin, **76**
bacterial infections, 180–181
baicalin, **65**
berberine, **46**

bulfalin, 112
buprenorphine, **12**
buspirone hydrochloride, **77**

caffeine, 44, **54**, 115–116
calcein, 56, 91, **136**, 146–147
camphor, 180–181
cannabidiol, **76**
capsaicin, **13**, 158
carbomer, 179
Carbopol, 179
carboxyfluorescein, 56, **135**, 146
carvacrol, 112
carveol, 118
carvone, 112, 113, 125
celecoxib, **63**
ceramides, 4–5, 118
    molecular structure, *6*
cetyltrimethylammonium bromide (CTAB),
    177–178, *178*, *179*
chemical penetration enhancers, 19–21
    modes of action, **21**
chloramphenicol, 56
cholesterol, 32, *34*
cimetidine, 56
1.8-cineole, 112, 113, 118, 119, 128, 155, 158,
    167, 180–181
cineole, 144
citral, 158, 167
citronellol, 124
clindamycin, 56
clonidine, **12**
cocamide diethanolamine, 158
coenzyme Q10 (Q10), **82**

208   Index

colchicin, **64**
confocal laser scanning microscopy
    (CLSM), 56–57
corneocytes, 3–4, 87
corneodesmosomes, 4
corticosteroids, 43
co-solvents, 118–119
curcumin, **46**, **53**, 56, 128, **136**, 151–152
cyclodextrin, 151
cyclosporine A, 44, **51**, **67**, 123, 131, **132**, *141*,
    171, **172**, *174*
cymene, 143

dapsone, 128, **137**
    as penetration enhancers, 158–159, *159*
deformable vesicles, 57, 109
deoxycholic acid (DA), 56–57
deoxyribonucleic acid (DNA), 56
dermal delivery, 8–13
    advantages of, 10–13
    target sites, 8–10, *9*
Dermaroller, *166*, 166–167, *168*
dermis, 2
dexamethasone, **60–61**
diazepam, 113, 144
diclofenac, **13**, **52**, **61–62**, 79
didodecyldimethyl ammonium bromide
    (DDAB), 177–178, *178*, *179*
differential scanning calorimetry (DSC), 90,
    111, 182–183
diflunisal, **63–64**
Dil, 177
1,2-dimyristoyl-sn-glycero-3-phosphocholine
    (DMPC), 56–57, 121
dioleoylphosphatidylcholine (DOPC), 32
dioleoylphosphatidylethanolamine (DOPE),
    32, 91
1,2-dioleoyl-sn-glycero-3-
    phosphoethanolamine-N-
    (lissamine rhodamineB), 169–170
dipalmitoylphosphatidylcholine (DPPC), 32
distearoylphosphatidylcholine (DSPC), 32, 91
distearoylphosphatidylethanolamine
    (DSPE), 32
1,2-distearoyl-snglycero- 3-phosphocholine
    (DSPC), 91–92
dithranol, 44
DOPE liposomes, 91
doxyl stearic acid (DSA), 182–183
drug delivery systems, liposomes as, **45–55**
drug lipophilicity, 114
drug permeation rate, 18

dyphylline, 44

edge activators, 57
elastic vesicles, 57, 109
electron spin resonance (ESR), 182–183
encapsulation efficiency (EE%), 123, 128
enoxacin, 36
eosinophilic pustular folliculitis, 156
epidermis, 2–8
epigallocatechin-3- gallate (EGCG), **67**
erectile dysfunction drugs, 160–161
erythromycin, **50**, **76**
Escherichia coli, 180–181
essential oils, 19
esters, 19
estradiol, **12**, 112, 113, 120, 143, 157
ethanol, 119–122
ethers, 19
ethinyl estradiol, **12**
ethosomes, 58, 72
    as dermal and transdermal drug delivery
    systems, **73–83**
etodolac, 113
eucalyptol, 112, 115
eugenol, 113, 124

Fahr, A., 109
farnesol, 112
fatty acids, 19
fenchone, 128, 143, 150, 151, 158, 167
fentanyl, **12**
ferulic acid, **135**, 148
fibroblast growth factor (bFGF), **48**
finasteride, 56, **73**, 124, 149–150
fisetin, **81–82**
flexible vesicles, 57, 109
fluorescein, 36
fluorescein isothiocyanate, 17
5-fluorouracil, 44, **65–66**, **82–83**, 112,
    113–114, 120
follicular penetration, 15–16, *16*
freeze fracture electron microscopy
    (FFEM), 86

geraniol, 112
giant unilamellar vesicles (GUV), 34
granisetron, **13**
growth hormone (hGH), **68**

hail follicles, 14–17
haloperidol, 112
heparin, 44

hepatitis B surface antigen (HBsAg), **69**, **79**
hexapeptide, **54**
hinokitiol, 120
hipodermis, 2
hydrocortisone, 44, **60**, 112, 120, 144
hydrophilic model drugs, 145–147
hydroxy propyl β-cyclodextrin (HPβCD), 151
hypertension, 178–179

ibuprofen, **78**, 112
idebenone, 126, **137**, **172**, 177
immunosuppressive drugs, 131, 141
indinavir, **77**
indomethacin, 112, 143, 144, 157
insulin, 57, **69**
intercellular route, 14–15
interferon, 44, 56
intracellular lipids, 4–5
intrafollicular penetration, 15–16, *16*
invasomes, 72, 109–190
    characterization of, 123–129
    development of, 109–111
    ethanol as penetration enhancer, 119–122
    fluidity of, 181–184
    mode of action, 184–186, *185*
    as nanocarriers for dermal and transdermal
        drug delivery, **132–140**
    particle size, 125
    as penetration enhancers, 129–161
        acne drugs, 158–159
        alopecia drugs, 159–160
        antihypertensive drugs, 152–156
        antioxidants, 148
        avanafil, 160–161, *161*
        curcumin, 151–152
        cyclosporine A, 131, 141
        dapsone, 158–159, *159*
        drugs for the management of prostatic
            hyperplasia, 149–151
        erectile dysfunction drugs, 160–161
        hydrophilic model drugs, 145–147
        isotretinoin, 156
        minoxidil, 159–160
        nonsteroidal anti-inflammatory drugs,
            156–158
        skin lighteners, 147–148
        temoporfin (mTHPC), 141–145
    with physical penetration enhancing
        method, 162–179, **163–165**
        massage, 169–170, *170*
        microneedles, 162–167
        ultrasound, 167–169

preparation of, 122–123
safety profile of, 187
structure and composition of, *110*
terpenes as penetration enhancers,
    111–119
therapeutic effectiveness of, 171–180
    acne, 176–178
    alopecia, 171, *174*
    anti-cancer therapy, 171–176, **172–173**
    bacterial infections, 180–181
    hypertension, 178–179
    photodynamic therapy, 171–176
    skin lightening, 179–180
iontophoresis, 57, 149–151
isotretinoin, 124, 125, 129, **139**, 156
isradipine, 153, **173**, 179–180, *180*

keratin, 3
keratinocytes, 14
keratohyalin, 3
ketones, 113, 143
ketoprofen, **62**, 157
kojic acid, 147

Labrasol, 72, 159
large unilamellar vesicles (LUVs), 34, 126
LeciPlex systems, 177–178, *178*, *179*
lecithin, 128
levonorgestrel, **12**, 120
lidocaine, **13**, 44, **59–60**, 112
limonene, 112, 113, 116–118, 119, 124, 125,
    128, 143–144, 145–147, 150–151,
    155, 157–158, 167
linalool, 112
lipid-protein-partitioning (LPP) theory, 20
lipophilic drugs, 143–144
lipophilicity, 114
liposomes, 31–35
    advantages of, 35
    classification, 34
    composition, 34, 35–36
    as drug delivery systems, 35,
        43–57, **45–55**
    mechanisms of action, **70**
        penetration of intact liposomes, 72–90
    physicochemical properties, 32,
        35–43, **37–42**
        influence of lipid composition, 35–36
        influence of particle size, 36
        surface charge, 36–43
    preparation, 35
    size of, 36

structure of, *33*
surface charge, 36–43
local depots, 43
long periodicity phase (LPP), *6*, 6–8

madecassoside, **49**
massage, 169–170, *170*
mechanical dispersion, 122
medium-sized unilamellar vesicles (MUV), 34
mefenamic acid, 118
melatonin, **77**
meloxicam, **63**
menthol, 112, 116–117, 180–181
menthone, 116–117, 118, 119
methotrexate, **50**
methylphenidate, **13**
microneedles, 162–167
midazolam, 143
minoxidil, **49**, **73**, **134**, 159–160
monoterpenes, 112
multilamellar large vesicles (MLV), 34
multivesicular vesicles (MVV), 34

naproxen, **52**, 116
nerolidol, 112, 116, 119, 125
nicotine, **12**, 18
nimesulide, 157
nitroglycerin, **12**, 18
non-steroidal anti-inflammatory drugs
        (NSAIDs), 58, 72, 156–158
norelgestromin, **12**
norethindrone, **12**

oleic acid, 115
oligolamellar vesicles (OLV), 34
olmesartan, 125, **138**, 153–154
oxide terpenes, 143
oxides, 113
oxybutynin, **12**
paeoniflorin, **82–83**
paeonol, **81**
papaverine hydrochloride, **70**
particle size
    invasomes, 125
    liposomes, 36
penetration enhancement, 19–21
    chemical penetration enhancers, 19–21
    lipid-protein-partitioning theory, 20
    methods, *20*
penetration enhancer-containing vesicles
        (PEVs), 34, 72, 159–160
peptide vaccine, **80**
Pharmasolve, 177

phenylethyl resorcinol, 147, 179–180, *181*
phosphatidyl glycerol (PG), 32
phosphatidyl inositol (PI), 32
phosphatidylcholine (PC), 32
phosphatidylethanolamine (PE), 32
phosphatidylserine (PS), 32
phosphodiesterase type 5 (PDE5)
        inhibitor, 160
phospholipids, *34*
Phospholipon, 144, 153
photodynamic therapy (PDT), 56, 171–176
physical penetration enhancing method,
        162–179, **163–165**
    massage, 169–170, *170*
    microneedles, 162–167
    ultrasound, 167–169
poly(d,l-lactic-co-glycolic acid) (PLGA), 16
polydispersity index (PDI), 124, 126, 177
polyvinylpyrrolidone (PVP)-iodine, **46**
progesterone, 36, 44
Propionibacterium acne, 178
propranolol, 112, 113, 143
propylene glycol, 118–119
prostatic hyperplasia, 149–151
psoralen, **51**
pulegone, 118
push effect, 121
pyrrolidones, 19

quercetin, **47**

regional delivery, 10, 19
resonance energy transfer (RET), 91
resveratrol, **48**
retinoid, 156
rezorcinol, **139**, **173**
rhodamine B, 17
rivastigmine, **12**
rose oxide, 118
rotigotine, **13**

safranal, 118
scopolamine, **12**
selegiline, **13**
sertraline, **69–70**
sesquiterpenes, 112, 114
short periodicity phase (SPP), 6
shunt route transport, 15
sildenafil, 154
skin, 2
    drug permeation rate, 18
    drug transport routes, 14–18
        intercellular route, 14–15

transappendageal transport, 15
transcellular route, 14
epidermis, 2–8
skin lighteners, 147–148, 179–180
small angle X-ray diffraction (SAXD), 116
small unilamellar vesicles (SUVs), 34, 126
Soluphor, 177
sorption promoters, 19–21
Staphylococcus aureus, 180–181
1-stearoyl-snglycero- 3-phosphocholine
        (stearoyl-LPC), 91
stratum basale, 2
stratum corneum, 2–8
    fluidity of lipid bilayers, 111
    penetration routes, *14*
    and properties of liposomes, 187
stratum granulosum, 2
stratum lucidum, 2
stratum spinosum, 2
subcutaneous layer, 2
sulphoxides, 19
surface charge, 36–43
surfactants, 19

tacrolimus, 44
tadalafil, 154
tamoxifen, **45**, 112
temoporfin (mTHPC), **54**, **66**, **78**, *120*, 123,
        126, 126–127, *127*, **133**, 141–145,
        142, 171, **172**, 174–176, *175*, 182
terbinafine hydrochloride (TH), **81**
terpenes, 19, 111–119, 143–144
    chemical structure of, *112*
    co-solvents, 118–119
    and drug lipophilicity, 114
    skin penetration enhancement by, 115–118
    structure-activity relationship, 113–114
testosterone, **12**, **74**
tetanus toxoid, **68**
tetracaine, **13**, 44, **59**
thermogravimetric analysis (TGA), 121
thymol, 143, 180–181
thyrotropin-releasing hormone (TRH), 119
tocopherol, **67**
tolterodine tartrate, 150–151
topical delivery, 9–10
transappendageal transport, 15
transcellular route, 14
Transcutol, 19, 72, 159, 177

transdermal drug delivery systems (TDDS), 8–13
    advantages of, 10–13
    aims of, 10
    defined, 10
    target sites, 8–10, *9*
    transfersomes, 58–72
transdermal products, **12–13**
transfersomes, 58–72, **59–71**, 85
transfollicular penetration, 15–16, *16*
transkarbams, 19
transmission electron microscopy (TEM), 86
tretinoin, 44, **49**
triamcinolone acetonide (TRMA), 43, 44
trihexyphenidyl hydrochloride (THP), 44, **74**

ultrasound, 167–169

valencene, 118
valsartan, 113
vardenafil, 128, 154–156
vesicles
    deformable, 57, 109
    elastic, 57, 109
    flexible, 57, 109
    giant unilamellar, 34
    large unilamellar, 34, 126
    mechanisms of action, 72–93, *84*
        penetration of intact vesicles, 72–90
        penetration of the drug released from
            vesicles, 93
        penetration-enhancing mechanism
            of, 90–93
        vesicle adsorption to and/or fusion
            with SC lipids, 90–93
    medium-sized unilamellar, 34
    multilamellar large, 34
    multivesicular, 34
    oligolamellar, 34
    penetration enhancer-containing, 34, 72,
        159–160
    small unilamellar, 34, 126
    as transdermal drug delivery
        systems, 57–72
viable epidermis, 3
vitamin A (retinoid), 156

wide angle X-ray diffraction (WAXD), 116

zidovudine, 112, 119